BE BEAUTIFUL SLIM & TRIM

By
AROONA REEJHSINGHANI

HEALTH HARMONY

Note from the Publishers

Any information given in this book is not intended to be taken as a replacement for medical advice. Any person with a condition requiring medical attention should consult a qualified practitioner or therapeutist.

BE BEAUTIFUL BE SLIM & TRIM

© Copyright with the Publisher

All rights are reserved. No part of this book may be reproduced, stored in a retrieval system or transmitted, in any form or by any means, mechanical, photocopying, recording or otherwise, without any prior written permission of the author.

Edition: 2006

Price: Rs. 75.00

Published by Kuldeep Jain for

HEALTH 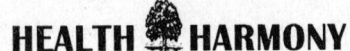 HARMONY
an imprint of
B. Jain publishers (P.) Ltd.
1921, Street No. 10, Chuna Mandi,
Paharganj, New Delhi 110 055 (INDIA)
Phones: 91-011-2358 0800, 2358 1100, 2358 1300
Fax: 91-011-2358 0471; Email: bjain@vsnl.com
Website: www.bjainbooks.com

Printed in India by:
J.J. Offset Printers

ISBN : 81-8056-202-6   BOOK CODE : BA-5652

CONTENTS

PART - I
BE BEAUTIFUL

A real beauty 1
Beauty is not skin deep 3
Tips for a radiant & healthy skin 5
Steps to a lovely skin 8
Save your skin 10
Look after your face 13
Combat a dry skin 15
Greasy skin - how to care 17
The ABC of haircare 19
Hair myths 23
Combat dandruff 25
Hairstyling 27
Hairstyle to suit your face 30
In house beauty treatments 32
Cure Black heads 35
Cure wWhite heads 37

Combat pimples 39
Hirsutism 41
Beautiful baby 44
Beauty after twenty 47
Teenage bBeauty 49
Beauty at thirty 51
Beauty at forty 53
Beauty at fifty 56
Beauty at 60 plus 59
Beat stress and rejuvenate yourself 62
Working woman's beauty care 64
Beauty hints for the working woman 66
Summer style 68
Be a winter beauty 73
ABC of monsoon beauty 75
How to make up 80
Cosmetic sins 83
Party beauty 85
Get more 87

PART - II
BE SLIM & TRIM

Introduction 91
Stay slim 93
Obesity 96
All about calories 98
Count your calories 100
Weight control 109

When exercising	112
Exercise therapy	114
Spot exercises	117
Whole body exercises	128
Light exercises	130
Fun exercises	132
Facial exercises	133
Increase body activity	136
Some myths about exercises	137
A good posture	139
Clothes to hide body defects	141
Colours and textures for obese people	144
Make-up secrets	146
You ask we answer	149
Combat bad eating habits	152
Distract yourself from food	154
7-Day menu for reducing	155

PART - 1
BE BEAUTIFUL

A Real Beauty

To be a real beauty one should be a winner in life, one should stand out amongst others and make an impression wherever one goes. Today beauty is not only external beauty but also inner beauty. To be really beautiful you have to live according to the laws of nature and believe in spirituality. Yukta Mookhey, the latest Miss World, lived according to these laws and she came out a winner. What are these laws?

Basically, these laws of nature teaches us to look at larger interests and nor just our own. You should be a vegetarian and non-alcoholic with spiritual inclinations. If you do not eat non-vegetarian food and do not imbibe liquor your mind will automatically have spiritual leanings. Vegetarian food increases Life, Purity, Health, Joy and Cheerfulness. Lord Krishna says in Bhagwat Gita that people who eat vegetarian food discover in themselves a secret strength which provides health and beauty. Vegetarian diet also has the power to reverse negative thought processes and life patterns. Vegetarian diet coupled with chanting Gayatri Mantra makes you a more assertive and vibrant person. Gayatri Mantra is the mantra used to invoke the Sun God. The worship of the Sun God is as old as the human race. Sun is known as the invincible God bestowed with eternal and timeless powers of blessing. Sun is the main source of life on this planet. He is the origin of life, feeling and thought and is the determining cause of existence of everything upon this earth. Luminous rays of the sun have the power of passing through the skin and being absorbed by the blood. The sun rays also destroy injurious toxins in the body and have great therapeutic properties. Therefore, Gayatri Mantra is of great value to a person who recites it regularly in the early morning sunlight after getting up from bed. Beauty is just not about body toning, shaping and weight loss but also about bringing the mind and body into harmony with each other so that you become an integrated personality emanating goodness and kindness for all creatures on this earth.

Gayatri Mantra

Om bhoor bhuvah suwah

Tat savitur vareniyum

Bhargo devasya deemahi

Dhiyo yo nah prachodayat

Cleansing the spirit and the body by chanting mantras makes the body not only beautiful externally but also spiritually.

Beauty is not Skin Deep

Beauty is not skin deep. A real beauty also has a beautiful soul within herself, which makes her kind and gentle. You must remember that besides having external beauty if you have a kind word and a helping hand, besides giving you inner serenity and outer beauty it will open wide the floodgates of goodwill and fellow feeling. Here are some home truths, if you will follow them faithfully you will spread goodwill and cheer all around you.

1. Never laugh at anyone's dreams.
2. Don't injure your relations because of a little dispute. Always think before you talk.
3. If you find an old person or a pregnant lady standing in a bus or a train offer your seat to them.
4. In the same way if you find a physically handicapped person or an old lady behind you in the queue, let them go ahead of you.
5. Someone will always be looking at you as an example of how to behave, don't let them down.
6. Give people more than they expect and do it cheerfully.
7. Don't be so concerned with your own ideas that you forget your manners.

8. Don't dismiss a good idea because you do not like the person who is giving it to you.

9. Never say anything uncomplimentary about your friends, your neighbors and your relations in front of others.

10. When you say the word a Sorry, mean it.

11. Never take anyone for granted and never let anyone take you for granted. Remember that no time spent with your elders, children and sick is wasted.

12. No matter how old you get, always hug and kiss your parents whenever you meet them to make them feel wanted and loved.

13. When talking to someone always have a pleasant voice. Even if your looks are just ordinary your voice will attract people. It is a great beauty asset. So cultivate a soft and gentle voice. Tone it with sincerity and polish it to a pleasing pitch and see that your conversation is always pleasant. Always be free from ugly gossip.

14. Never befriend someone you love, always befriend a person who loves you.

Tips for a Radiant & Healthy Skin

Here are a few tips; if you follow them diligently you will not only have a radiant skin but also well-being and vitality.

1. Junk food : This food which is overloaded with salt, sugar, fats and spices slows down the flow of important and essential juices which adversely affects the skin and gives rise to embarressing skin blemishes. Therefore, you should always eat wholesome meals, simply cooked or not cooked at all with plenty of cereals, moderate amount of proteins and as much of fresh vegetables and fruits as you can eat.

2. Salt and sugar : They are white poisons and should be eaten to the barest of minimum. They not only increase your weight but are also enemies of a clear skin. White sugar contains no vitamins and minerals. Sugar in any form like sweets, desserts, chocolates, pastries, cakes, ice cream, etc. not only give rise to diseases but are fattening and harmful for the skin. Similarly, salt is harmful to the skin. It encourages water retention and therefore puffiness of the skin. It should not be taken more than 2.3 gm daily which is the recommended daily intake.

3. Use steamed and grilled food : Avoid fried food. Instead grill, roast or bake food. If you want to eat fried foods then

cut them into large pieces and fry them at high temperature so that food is fried quickly and therefore absorbs less oil. Pat off the excess oil with paper towels.

4. Drink plenty of water : Water is the nector of life. Drink 8 to 10 glasses of water daily. This not only prevents constipation which gives rise to a sluggish skin but also puts a sparkle in your complexion and clear the blood stream of all the impurities.

5. Sleep : Get enough sleep in the night. If you have a sound sleep the body gets a chance to renew itself and decaying cells are eliminated through metabolic process. Average adult needs 8 to 10 hours of sleep daily. Less hours of sleep can result in under eye dark circles, dead skin and disease like high blood pressure, besides it is a scientific fact that it shortens life considerably.

6. Take time for prayer and meditation : Meditation is of tremendous value for maintaining mental and spiritual health. Prayer and meditation are food for the soul, strength and beauty for the body.

7. Junk food reduces the most important mineral in our body, namely zinc. It is needed for the production of the new healthy cells on the skin. Therefore, eat some nuts and seeds daily which are a good source of zinc.

8. Intense heat and cold : These have bad effect on the skin. Heat has a drying effect on the skin. As the natural oils begin to dry the skin starts to wrinkle and brown spots appear on it. In hot weather therefore you should moisturize your skin regularly to replenish lost moisture and natural oils.

As heat so the cold. Both make the skin dry and rough. Intense cold gives the skin a flaky appearance and hastens the appearance of thread viens on the cheeks. Again moisturizing the skin regularly prevents the skin from going bad.

9. Swimming in the salt water is good for the skin but you should immediately wash off the salt water with fresh water, otherwise the salt will make the skin dry and produce burning and itching. If your skin is extremely dry, you should never wash it with tap water because the salts and calcium in the water will make it drier, therefore always wash with mineral water. Never wash your face with hard water. Use softening substances like bath salts for bathing.

10. Air conditioners dry up the skin, so you should always apply a good moisturising cream - every night. Always remove make up in the night before going to sleep and make it scrupulously clean so that the cells have a chance to renew themselves.

Steps to a Lovely Skin

1. Keep out of the sun as much as possible especially between 12 to 4 in the afternoon when the sun is at its highest. Whenever you go out in the suns use a sunscreen of SPF 15. And always wear sunglasses to protect your eyes from getting tiny wrinkles. Always apply moisturizer twice a day whether you have a normal, dry or greasy skin. Moisturizer seals in the natural moisturizer of the skin, softens the surface of the skin and plumps out the fine lines.

2. Before sleeping in the night, remove all your make-up especially eye makeup with a creamy eye make-up remover. This will not only remove dryness around the eyes but will also help prevent crow's feet. After removing dirt and make-up, wash your face and pat dry. Finish the routine with a rich nourishing cream to seal in the moisture and to provide the necessary oils to beautify the skin.

3. Eat a diet rich in vegetables and fruits. Every day you should eat at least 1 medium apple. 1 cup raw leafy vegetables, ½ cup either chopped raw vegetable juice, ¼ cup dried fruits. The above mentioned diet will provide you with calcium, fibre, folic acid, iron, potassium, magnesium, beta-carotene and Vitamins B-2, C, E and K. These all are essentials of a healthy diet which are very essential for maintaining a healthy skin and body. You must always eat a variety of at

least 5 fruits and vegetables per day.

4. Drink plenty of water and fruit juices to detoxify the body.
5. Maintian a constant weight by doing regular exercises and avoid alcohol, smoking and drugs.
6. Be gentle with your skin. Rubbing or pinching the skin promotes fine lines and encourages wrinkles.
7. Always go in for cold showers rather than hot baths. Cold showers tone the skin and stimulate the nervous system.
8. Avoid unnecessary facial expressions like blinking, staring, scowling, frowning as these will leave an indelible mark on your face making you look ugly. Always try to cultivate a happy and cheerful outlook so that you always look cheerful. Cheerfulness is a beauty asset which always attracts people.

If you follow all the above steps diligently you will be a healthy and a happy person. So remember don't ever frown. You never know who is falling in love with your smile.

■

Save Your Skin

The skin is the largest organ of the human body. It is composed of cells which keep dying and being renewed every day. The skin is that part of body that most easily exhibits the effects of abuse and neglect. It is the mirror of your health, both physical and mental, therefore it is a perfect meter by which you can judge the state of a person's health.

The skin consists of two layers. The top layer is called epidermis and beneath this we have dermis which is a jelly-like substance supported by bundles of collagen fibers and below this there is a layer of fat. As you grow older the circulation of blood to the skin decreases and it loses its youthful appearance, its colour changes and wrinkles begin to oppear on its surface. The speed of ageing starts at 25. It is slow between 30 to 35, fast between 35 to 50 and very quick between 50 to 65. But you can cheat the calendar and preserve your youth by giving your skin regular care and attention from within and without.

Lack of proper circulation of blood to the skin is mostly due to lack of proteins, vitamins D and C. Protein foods supply all the amino-acids essential for keeping your skin youthful. If the proteins are inadequate in the body the tissues begin to sag causing wrinkles to appear. Like proteins, vitamins are important for rebuilding of the tissues and muscles of the face and body and prevention of wrinkles. Between the cells of the skin is a cementing substance know as collagen which depends upon vitamin C for its elasticity. Always remember that your facial muscles are living elastic tissues and that they can be nourished and built up from inside only with a good and healthy diet, and regular care of the skin. More often it is the commercially sold beauty products which are loaded with chemicals which make the complexion burn, itch, sting and turn swollen and red. Worse still we should learn to know our skin type and give it a tailor-made regime which suits our skin type rather by following blindly what is followed by our friends, by film stars or what is shown on. T.V. An easy way to discover what type of skin you have is to wipe your face with a dry tissue when you get up from bed in the morning. If there is oil on the tissue then you have a greasy skin, if there is grease only in the central panel then you have a combination skin, and if there is no grease on the tissue then you have a dry skin. To check a dry face wash it with soap and water, if your skin feels stretched or too tight then you have a dry skin and if your skin feels smooth and supple then you have a normal skin.

The first step towards maintaining a good skin is cleansing. Clean your face both morning and night with a good cleansing cream.

After cleansing comes toning. Toning removes greasiness, closes pores, refines the skin and it gives the skin a smooth, clean texture which can hold make-up for long hours. For a dry skin, skin toner is used and for a greasy skin astringent is used. Take a small piece of cotton, dip it in cold water, squeeze it between your fingers and then pour toner or astringent on it and apply it on your face, this way the cotton will absorb less lotion.

After toning comes nourishment. Every type of skin needs a moisturizer. Apply moisturizer after cleaning and toning the skin. Moisturizer rejuvenates the skin by making it more supple and beautiful.

∎

Look after Your Face

Your skincare facial routine is the key to your drop dead looks. Unless your facial skin is glossy, young and beautiful no amount of make-up can help you look beautiful. To maintain a beautiful skin you must follow a daily skin care routine.

Cleansing

Whether you have a dry, normal, oily or a combination skin you have to keep it scrupulously clean always. You should never use soap on the face because it not only dries up the skin but sometimes its chemical can do more harm than good to the skin. Always use a good cleansing milk. Apply the cleanser in circular upward movements using your fingertips for cream cleanser and cotton wool for liquid cleanser. Remove eye make up gently with cotton wool pads soaked in eye make up remover. Remove mascara by placing a moistened tissue under the lower lashes and stroking both sets of lashes together with cotton wool pads soaked in the cleanser.

Washing

Wash your face with light circular movements. Rinse your face thoroughly and then pat dry with a soft towel.

Toner

Skin toners are very refreshing and their evaporating and

cooling action couses the pores to shrink temporarily. Toners act as additional cleaners for oily skins and also remove any traces of grease left behind by the cleanser. The mildest forms of toners are called freshners or delicate toners. Astringents are stronger then toners and are used on very greasy skins. They should not be used on dry skins or on dry areas or combination skins.

Immediately after cleaning the face, apply a small amount of toner or astringent on the face.

Moisturizer

A moisturizing cream should follow the toner. It helps to offset the evaporating effects of the sun, wind, air conditioning and environmental pollution. It helps in protecting the skin by sealing in the vital natural moisture of the skin. It also acts as a perfect base for any type of makeup. Smooth the moisturizer over the face in upward circular movements with your fingertips, being careful not to drag the skin.

If you follow the skin routine daily, you will have a lovely and a beautiful skin which will look attractive and beautiful even without make-up.

■

Combat a Dry Skin

Dry skin is a very delicate skin which if left untreated gives rise to premature wrinkling of the skin. Dry skin is the first sign of Vitamia A deficiency. Therefore if you are suffering from a dry skin you should take vitamin A capsules of 25,000 units per day for 2 weeks and then you should go in for maintenance level of 10,000 to 20,000 units daily. If your diet seems to be sufficient in vitamin A, which means that you are regularly eating carrots, sweat potatoes, and liver, then dry skin may be a result of inadequate unsaturated oils. Try adding 2 tablespoons of oil in your soup, rise or dal.

Do's & Dont's for Dry Skin

1. If you have dry skin then use a glycerine or a super fat soap on the body.
2. After bathing do not rub your skin, instead pat your skin dry with a soft towel to reduce irritation of the skin. Dry yourself nicely after taking your bath, if water is left to evaporate on the skin it dries up the skin further.
3. Apply moisturizer immediately after drying the skin. It puts a waterproof layer between the skin and the air thereby preventing moisture loss.
4. Never, never use soap on the face and neck if you have a dry skin. Instead take 1 tablespoon warm milk and add to it a pinch of turmeric and few drops of oil. Dip a piece of

cotton in it and clean the skin. You will be amazed to find that it removes more dirt than any cleanser in the market and at the same time makes the skin soft and smooth.

5. After cleansing the skin pat a thin film of oil over the surface to seal in the moisture.

6. Never use an astringent on a dry skin.

7. Deep cleanse the skin once a week by steaming it, since steam encourages the secretion of natural sebum.

8. Vaseline or petroleum jelly is the best bet for a dry skin. But before using any greasy preparation on the skin, always use a moisturizer first. At night remove your make up with a cleansing milk. After removing the make up wipe with skin tonic and then massage in nourishing cream. After half an hour remove the skin tonic and apply moisturizer. If you are using commercial creams change them time to time because the skin needs a change of preparation just as our body needs change of air.

Vinegar makes an ideal skin tonic. The skin has an acid mantle and vinegar being acidic restores this. Always use one part of vinegar to 8 parts of water. This also prevents itchiness during winter and the tight feeling a dry skin has after it has been washed.

Here is a simple but effective skin tonic. Put 3 tablespoons of dried mint leaves in 2 cups water. Boil for 3 minutes. Strain and put in 2 cups vinegar. Apply on your face with cotton wool. The vinegar helps restore the acid mentle of the skin.

Always use a sunscreen whenever going out. This must have the SPF or sun protection factor written on it. The SPF is the protecting power of the sun screen.

Greasy Skin - How to Care

Greasy skin looks shiny, thick, slightly toneless, has coarse pores, pimples and other blemishes. An oily skin has excess oil or sebum which sometimes blocks the pores. If this oily blockage is not removed it hardens and white heads are formed. The whiteheads become blackheads when it gets oxidized by air. And if these are not taken care of then you get hard bumps under the skin which turn into pus filled pimples.

Vitamin B helps in checking the extra oil secretion of the skin. Brewers yeast tablets work wonders on a greasy skin. Add brewers yeast to your daily diet. This invaluable B vitamin will normalize the oil balance on the skin. Liver also helps in checking the oiliness of the skin if taken a few times in a week. Also eat plenty of fresh fruits and vegetables. Pork, fried and highly seasoned foods should be avoided and the diet should be restricted in fluids, sugar and salt.

Cleansing

Wash your face often with tap water and then pat dry. Here is a good cleanser. Put a teaspoon of skimmed milk in a cup, add a pinch of haldi and enough water to create a milky consistency. Apply with cotton wool all over your face and neck and then remove with facial tissue and blot dry.

In the night before going to sleep clean the face with cleansing milk and then apply astringent. Astringent will not only close the pores but will also regulate the sebaceous secretions.

In the morning, clean your face and then apply this refresher. Mix together lemon juice, water and cumber juices in equal quantities. Strain through a fine cloth. Freeze in the ice cube tray. Just run an ice cube lightly over your face, dry it under the fan and you will not only feel a cool tingling feeling but this will also alleviate the oily skin condition considerably.

You should steam your face at lease once a week. But you should not take steam for more than 1 minute. Now make a facial with brewers yeast. Mix one teaspoon each of yeast and milk powder with water to make a loose paste. Apply to a freshly cleaned skin that has been rinsed with water containing a few drops of apple cider vinegar. Let it dry completely and then rinse it. Every skin requires nourishing cream whether it is dry or greasy. Apply the cream, leave it on for 15 minutes and then remove with astringent. Astringent closes and tightens the pores. Also you can remove the extra grease with sprit of camphor.

■

The ABC of Haircare

A   Is for Average number of hair on the head. Every human being has approximately one thousand hair roots. Each hair root grows through cycles. It grows for 3 to 5 years then it rests for 3 to 5 months and then sheds off. On an average there is a fall of 30 to 40, hair normally but if there is more hair fall then you should seek treatment. The hair fall is more than normal when you are washing you hair, so you need not worry if you see more hair coming out when you are shampooing it.

B   Is for Baldness which is due to a number of conditions. Poor diet is one of the main causes. Other causes are hereditary, prolonged illnesse of certain types like typhoid, pregnancy, menopause, etc., too much exposure to sun and an unclean scalp. A diet rich in Iron, Iodine and B vitamins can help grow hair on bald spots.

C   Is for Conditioner. Use conditioner sparingly. Don't slather it on because then it will make the hair look flat. Don't apply conditioner right from the roots, instead apply it about 5 inches from the roots, this will give the hair body as well as the bounce.

D   Is for Dandruff, which is very dangerous if not controlled. There are too types of dandruff, oily and dry. Oily dandruff is more dangerous than dry one. Do get your scalp treated immediately for dandruff.

E Is for Eating the right type of food, fruits and veggies either as salads or in the form of juices. They can put the bounce and lights back into your hair.

F Is for Fine hair. This type of hair is generally limp and tends to cling close to the head. The best remedy for this type of hair is this : Take 1 egg, 2 table spoons castor oil, 1 teaspoon each of vinegar and glycerine. Mix together in the electric blender. Massage into the scalp. Wash off after half an hour. This will not only give body to the hair but will also make it look thicker and shiny.

G Is for Gel. You should avoid using gels. If at all you use them they should be the non-alcoholic ones, the ones containing alcohol dry up the hair.

H Is for hygiene. With pollution almost reaching threatening levels, you should try to wash your head daily, if not daily at least thrice a week to keep your scalp free from ailments and your hair clean.

I Is for inheritance. Good, shining, smooth and dark hair is inherited in seventy percent of cases. Baldness, thinning and greying hair are inherited from your parents, and you can do nothing about it.

J Is for Jealousy-worry, anxiety, hatred and mistrust. These pay havoc with emotional and physical health. Good thoughts are helpful allies towads maintaining hair beauty.

K Is for Keeping away from medicated shampoos. The medicated dandruff removing shampoos don't clear the dandruff but make it return with a vengeance. These give only temporary relief. These dandruff chasers can do a staggering amount of scalp and hair damage.

L   Length of hair. Maximum length of hair which can grow is 70-90 cms.

M   Medicated hair oils; never use them because these contain white oil which leads to premature greying. For the same reason don't use hair dyes. They not only contain harmful chemicals which are harmful for the scalp and skin but if once discontinued will give you a full head of grey hair. They also cause premature baldness.

N   Is for Never using soap on the hair. Soap is very damaging to hair because it leaves an insoluble alkaline film on the scalp even after the hair has bean thoroughly rinsed. This deposit can close the oil openings in the scalp and its drying qualities may give rise to ugly dandruff, therefore, it is always wise to wash with a good shampoo.

O   Is for Oil: Oil in its natural form like pure coconut, olive oil or almond oil can do wonders for your hair. You can give a thorough oil massage to your hair once a week to keep them from drying out.

P   Is for Pert bobs or layered cuts. These are the rosiest things today. These hair styles are considered sleek and manageable. Career woman and collegians are opting for short hair because these make them look stylish and gives them a cool image. Some are even going for tonsured look. Many youngsters are going around with smoothly shaven scalps.

Q   Is for Quality. To maintain quality hair sensibly keep a healthy scalp by shampooing it regularly with natural ingredients with shikakai, ritha, amla, henna, etc.

R   Is for Rubbing your hair vigorously with a towel. This may harm its structure. Instead wind the towel around the head and let it dry.

S   Is for split ends. Split ends are the result of excessive use of bleaching, dyeing, tinting, hair dryers and curlers. Split ends should be trimmed every two months to avoid further separation of hair layers.

T   Is for Travelling. Whenever you are travelling tie your hair. Windblown hair not only look untidy but also tend to tangle and attract dust and grime. When you reach your destination you can untie your hair.

U   Is for Untidy hair. Always keep your hair tidy and good looking. One way of achieving this is to rinse your hair after shampooing with 2 tablespoons vinegar or a juice of lime diluted in warm water. This gives the hair softness, brightness and a healthy look.

V   Is for Very oily hair. To treat an oily scalp, wash your hair with multani mitti and warm water. Soak a big lump of multani mitti in a vessel of warm water. When it softens add juice of a lime. Rub this into the scalp and leave for half an hour and then wash off. This not only removes extra oil from the hair but makes them soft and thick.

W   Is for Warm weather. Hair grows faster in warm weather than in cold weather. Female hair grows slower than male hair.

X   Is Xtra-terrestrial. Which is what you look like when you go overboard with your hair accessories.

Y   Is for You; remember to go in for a style which suits your age and not which suits your daughter.

Z   For Zest in life; worries and stress will not only make your life miserable but will also make your hair fall like feathers.

Hair Myths

1. *Myth* - Oil helps hair grow faster.

   Fact - Hair grows from the follicle beneath the scalp and the oil does not in any way effect the growth of hair. But when you massage the hair with oil, the massage helps to increase the blood flow to the hair follicles and this in turn increases the hair growth. This shows that not oil but massage helps in the growth of hair.

2. *Myth* - The more frequently you cut your hair the faster it will grow.

   Fact - Hair grows only 1 cm every 15 days and no amount of cutting will change this. However split ends will not attack your hair if you trim it regularly every 3 months.

3. *Myth* - Split ends interfere with hair growth.

   Fact - Split ends do not it any way effect the growth of hair since the hair grows from the follicles from within the scalp.

   Split ends occur when the cuticle is damaged and the fibres of the cortex unravel. Dry and brittle hair only splits at the end and this can only be cured by regularly trimming the hair.

4. *Myth* - Colouring the hair regularly will alter the natural pigmentation of hair.

   Fact - Colouring is done only on the hair and the new growth of hair comes back with your natural pigmentation.

If the opposite was true you will never need retouching.

5. *Myth* - Oil can cure dandruff.

   Fact - Oil applied before washing of hair interferes with cleaning the hair properly. This results in dandruff. Oil plays just the opposite role, it increases dandruff instead of reducing it.

6. *Myth* - if you pull out a grey hair, you will get two grey hair in its place.

   Fact - Only 1 hair grows out from one follicle, so how can two hair grow out from one follicle?

7. *Myth* - Beer is good for hair.

   Fact - Beer is very harmful for the hair. It not only gives rise to dandruff, but also dulls the hair and dries the scalp.

8. *Myth* - Shaving the head will help in the hair growth.

   Fact - Only one hair grows out of a follicle. Shaving or no shaving, the hair will remain as before.

■

Combat Dandruff

Dandruff is the disorder of the scalp which appears in the form of little white flakes in your hair. It is usually accompanied by an itchy, scratchy feeling in the head. Dandruff mostly effects the head either in the rainy season or in the winter months. Most of the people suffer from dandruff sometimes in their lives. In ordinary cases it can be removed with home treatment only, but in persistent and chronic cases you should seek medical advice. Here we are dealing with ordinary cases of dandruff.

Dandruff can give rise to acne and pimples. A little dandruff sloughing off your head is not harmful but if too much of it settles on the scalp, harmful bacteria begin to multiply. These are held back due to excessive oil in the scalp which results in itching and ringworm of the scalp. If this germ laden dandruff falls on your back and shoulders, it gives rise not only to acne but also red itchy patches which keep on spreading. The best way to keep away from dandruff is to wash your hair daily. This will help remove grime and help your hair to be free from dandruff.

Dandruff can also lead to baldness, therefore even if it is very mild it should be dealt with immediately.

Remedies

1. For dry dandruff the best remedy is to mix lime juice with egg white and massage into the scalp. Leave for half an hour and then wash off.

2. For very scaly and itchy scalp Vitamin E oil liberally into the scalp. Cover with scarf and go to bed. In the morning wash your head either with shikakai or baby shampoo and rinse the hair afterwards either with 2 tablespoons apple cider vinegar or lime juice dissolved in 2-3 mugs of water. Do this twice a week till the itching and scabs disappear.

3. Another good anti-dandruff shampoo is made by beating yolks of 2 eggs in ½ cup of warm water. Massage this into the scalp and hair thoroughly. Rinse carefully and then use a final rinse of 2 tablespoons of apple cider vinegar mixed in water.

4. Supplement your diet with B vitamins. Take yeast tablets, eat liver frequently and take plenty of fresh fruits, vegetables and protein rich foods.

5. Never use the "medicated dandruff shampoos", so widely advertised. These medicated dandruff shampoos do not clear the dandruff but make it return with a vengeance. These give only temporary relief. These dandruff chasers which are being widely advertised can do a staggering amount of scalp and hair damages, therefore always go in for natural means to control your dandruff.

   If you eat the right food comprising of fresh fruits, vegetables and juices and keep your scalp clean you will never fall prey to dandruff.

Hairstyling

Your hairstyling should be unique and so much attractive that others should want to copy it. The hair should be smooth, soft and shimmering and the style should suit you, something trendy yet unique. Besides the styling, hair colour is definitely the fashion of the millennium. The colour should be bright, shiny and dark.

Styles:

1. Most of the international magazines have predicted that long hair will be the rage in the new millennium, but if you want, you can perm your hair for a change because straight hair has been in fashion for a long, long time.
2. If you do not want to perm your hair you can curl your hair temporarily. It is done with tons and sometimes the effect is better then a perm.
3. Besides you can go in for hair jewels which are winning many fans because they are inexpensive, versatile and just plain fun.
4. During hot summer days, a few tiny clips in right places can prevent a bad hair day.
5. A headband can tidy up beach battered locks and a rhinestone barrette can turn a daytime look glittery enough for a night party.

6. The newest trend in hair jewellery are the round crystals on a snap which look like they are literally floating on the hair.
7. And the freshest style is twisting chunks of hair in baby-sized jaw clips and mixing headbands with bobby pins.

But before going in for hair ornaments, you should keep your age in view. Women in the twenties and thirties should go in for headbands and clips whilst preteens should go in for snaps on accessories in the shape of butterflies, flowers, frogs, sea horses, dragonflies or butterfly tremblers, butterflies that tremble when you move. These tremblers have become very popular in the international fashion scene. Besides keeping your age in mind you should select the ornament with great care. A good ornament can make your look very stylish, but a badly chosen one can end up making you look like a Christmas tree. Here are some hints to follow when you shop for hair ornaments.

1. A long feather in natural shade will look lovely if stuck in a pony tale or a chignon.
2. For a party you can slick back a low pony tail and poke several small feathers around the base of the rubber band.
3. If you buy baby clips go in for black or metallic colours only. Clips covered by fake flowers or multi-coloured plastic beads look kirsch. Scrunches should be bought in pastel colours rather than loud garish colours. For casual outings, you can decorate your hair with little combs in black, silver or gold.
4. Head scarves (full head coverings) should be made of knit, mohair and suede and should be delicately embroidered.

5. Necklaces, headbands, stones or chains that drape onto a persons forehead should also be very delicately made to make you look attractive and alluring and not somebody who has just walked out of circus.

■

Hairstyle to Suit Your Face

Your hair style should be unique and so attractive to make others want to copy you. Not only your hair should be smooth, soft and shimmering but the style should suit you. It should be trendy yet unique. Now checkout your facial shape and adopt the hairstyle that suits you. The right kind of hair style can make a tremendous difference to your appearance and personality. Style your hair according to the shape of your face. To find out the right shape of your face, tie your hair back with a valba band. Tie your hair back with a valba band, close one eye and outline your face shape with the help of a lipstick tube on the mirror in front of you.

Long face- Try to get a fringe this will shorten your face. Style hair fairly close to the top of the head combined with fullness at the sides. The hair should end either at the chin or the shoulders.

Round face- The hair should be fluffed at the crown and flattened at the sides which will provide more length to the face.

Diamond face- This type of face is broadest at the ears and check bones and narrow at the lower part of the face. The hair should be styled on the forehead with less volume at the top and the side slaving it longer at the nape.

Square face- The hair should be lifted off the forehead and come forward to the sides and jaw to create an illusion of narrowness and softness to the face. Have a soft perm to create body and soft jawline. Don't keep hair off the face.

Heart-shaped face - Decrease the width of the forehead and increase the width of the lower part of the face by getting a bob ending at the jawline. Get a light perm if you have hair of the shoulder length. A center parting with a fringe will add softness to the jawline.

Oval-shaped face. This the perfect shape and just about any style will suit this type of face.

Besides right hairstyle you can camouflage the facial defects with a hair style. If you have low forehead, style should be never brushed forward in bangs but to camouflage a high forehead get a fringe. If you have a long nose avoid center parting and always have long hair, short hair tend to make the nasal pores prominent. But if you have a short nose always wear your hair short and have some hair brushed across your forehead. For a projecting chin have a close cut at the crown and leave the hair linger at the nape. Also for a receding chin have long hair.

A right type of hair style will work wonders for you.

■

In House Beauty Treatments

Instead of wasting your time and money in a beauty saloon you can do the same treatments at home yourself with less than one-fourth the amount of money you spend in a saloon.

Facial

Facial is a sort of guardian angel which in a short time rejunuvates the skin. Tie up your hair. Then clean your face with a good cleansing milk. Wipe off with a piece of cottonwool dipped in water. Release impurities by steaming. Steaming is done by putting your face over a basin full of hot water, with a towel over your head to keep the steam in as long as possible. Steam for 5 minutes only. Hold your face 25 cms above the water otherwise you will have broken veins. For dry skin steam for 5 minutes and if you have oily skin then steam for 10 minutes. The heat dilates the pores and empties them of dirt and cleanses the skin of all its impurities. Thoroughly wipe with a damp napkin and pat dry. Now apply a facial scrub. Use gentle circular movements and avoid the eye areas. After 20 minutes wash off and apply a mask for greasy skin. Gently apply eye cream. After 20 minutes wash off and apply a alcohol free toner. While the skin is still damp apply a moisturizer.

Warning - Do not give yourself a facial if you have acne or other skin conditions. You might make the condition worse.

Perfect eyebrows

Only one professional brow-shaping done in a saloon can help you maintain perfect eyebrows all your life. Every day see your eyebrows in a mirror kept near an open window where you get plenty of light. If you see any stray hair just pluck them out with a tweezer. If you find that tweezing is painful then take the sting out of the operation by dabbing the eyebrows with a piece of cotton wool dipped either in eau-de-cologne or astringent lotion. All the stray hair from above the nose should be plucked out regularly by using a pair of scissors. This should be done daily without fail to keep your eyebrows permanently in shape.

Waxing

To prepare your own wax at home, take 250 grams of sugar and squeeze in juice of 6 large limes. Cook the mixture over gentle fire till it turns light brown and sticky. Remove from fire and mix in 1 tablespoon glycerine. Apply the wax in the direction of the hair growth with the help of a blunt knife. Press a clean strip of cotton cloth over the wax. Grip the edge of the strip firmly. Pull off in one swift motion against the skin in the opposite direction making the removal of hair easier. Before starting waxing on any area, dust the area with talcum powder to ensure that the wax pulls off cleanly. After waxing, moisturize the skin with a moisturizing lotion or cream.

Manicure

Your nails deserve a weekly manicure to keep them in a good condition. Remove old nail polish a day in advance to give them a chance to breathe in oxygen and to get the benefits of sun and air. Before beginning your manicure, wash your hands thoroughly with hot soapy water using a soft shaving brush. Apply cuticle remover over cuticles with a cotton bud. Cuticle remover softens and loosens cuticles. Never cut cuticles and do not push them back too hard as you might hurt live tissues at the nail base. Wash fingertips again, work off dead skin with a napkin and then dry hands thoroughly. Massage a little warm olive oil around the nails and then wipe thoroughly so that no trace of grease remains. Cut nails and shape them using a nail file. Use long movements in one direction. Gently level the tips with downward strokes so as to seal together the nail layers. Now scrub nails downwards with a nail brush dipped in warm soapy water and dry thoroughly. Place your hands firmly on a table and apply a thin even layer of nail polish. Stroke brush down the middle, base to tips and then do the sides. Stop and dry and apply a second thin coat and wait till it dries up. Finally apply a thin top coat and leave to dry. Reapply every few days sealing the edges to make your manicure last longer. Keep nail polish in the fridge to prevent it from thickening. Do not shake the nail polish bottle if you want to use it (it creates air bubbles). Roll between your palms instead.

Pedicure

Don't ever have long toe nails... It's just not done. Keep nails upto the edge of the toe. Cut straight across to prevent ingrown toe nails. File the nails carefully and remove old nailpolish. Push back cuticles with cottonbuds. Soak the feet in warm soapy water and scrub with a foot brush to remove dead cells. Dry well and nip off any ugly nails or bits of dead skin with scissors. Before applying nail polish, place small swabs of cotton between each toe. Paint the nails using a thin coat first and then follow up with 2 more coats of nail polish.

Cure Black Heads

Black heads are mostly caused by overactive sebaceous glands which produce excess oil. The oil comes up through the pores and if there is dirt or grime blocking the pores a bump forms under the skin. This hardens into a plug, the top of which when oxidized by air turns black and forms into black heads.

Ways to cure black heads

1. Make a good lather of 1 tablespoon grounded almonds and water and gently work this foam over the face. Then use a shaving brush to clean the face and open clogged pores. Take care not to use the brush too energetically or you will irritate your skin. Wash off with ordinary tap water.
2. A good cleansing of a very oily skin is a very effective measure in combating blackheads. A good cleanser for oily skin is ¼ cup shavings of baby soap, ¼ cup maize flour and ¼ cup grounded almonds. Put them in a container and use daily. Every day take a small amount in your hands and add enough water to make a smooth paste. Apply with a moistened shaving brush over your skin especially where the black heads are concentrated. This action will help to dislodge the embedded dirt and oil which are breeding ground of blackheads. Rinse the face in warm and then cold water. As a final rinse use a tablespoon of vinegar to a

cup of water and splash on the face.

Tomatoes are very useful when treating blackheads. The acid in the tomatoes thoroughly cleanses the skin thus keeping it free from clogged pores. Mash a tomato and strain through a fine sieve. Mix with grounded oatmeal and apply on the face. Leave on for 20 minutes and then wash off with tap water. You can also mix the paste with either curd or honey. You can also rub a slice of tomato over the place where you get blackheads with good results.

4. Besides, include vitamin A in your diet. Lack of this vitamin can create dead cells below the surface of the skin which clogs the oil glands and pores and prevents the normal lubrication of the skin.

5. If numerous large and closely grouped superficial blackheads are present, you can remove them by taking an ordinary piece of adhesive plaster. Heat the plaster and apply firmly on the portion where you have blackheads in the night, in the morning pull them off with a sharp tug. This if properly used is very effective in removing blackheads. This procedure may be repeated, but it should not be used on sensitive and dry areas. After reaming the plaster, dab on the skin a moisturizing lotion or cream.

■

Cure White Heads

White heads are tiny cysts which are formed due to the improper elimination of oil secreted from the grease glands. They have the appearance of hard white spots and they appear on any part of the body, but they are most commonly seen on the areas around the face especially around the nose, cheeks, temples and forehead. They mostly appear when you do not take care of your skin; therefore every time you apply makeup, remove it very nicely with good cleansing milk. Every time you come home from outside, clean your face with antiseptic soap and plenty of water. Do not use too much oil on the head. Even if you cannot do without oiling your hair, do not keep oil in your hair for more than 10 to 15 minutes. Also be vary of dandruff. It is the main culprit for giving rise to white heads. White head is beginning of a pimples.

Ways to cure white heads

1. A whitehead can be best removed by steaming the face for 1-2 minutes. When the whiteheads in the pores have softened, prick the apex with a clean sterilized needle. Then very gently press it out with your two fingers keeping them on either side of the whitehead and gently putting pressure

on it. Another way to remove whiteheads is to take shavings of baby soap and mix in table salt. Take a wet and soft face brush, dip in the mixture and very gently rub in the portions having white heads with the brush for a couple of minutes. Then wash off after a few rubbings. The whiteheads can be removed by gently pressing them out. But never let your fingernails press the skin and never squeeze the skin. This can cause scars and broken veins.

■

Combat Pimples

Pimples is a common disease amongst young people. In the beginning there are sebaceous plugs (known as black heads and white heads) in the sebaceous glands. Usually the infection causes the inflammatory process and the pimples set in. Red boils are formed and the size varies from a small seed to that of a pea. Initially they last for a few weeks then disappear leaving a temporary pigmentation. With recurring infections these boils develop into an abscess leaving behind unsightly scars.

Ways to cure pimples

1. The best remedy for pimples is your own spit. The spit found in your mouth early in the morning and midnight is very poisonous which kills the pimples. Every time you wake up in the night apply your spit on the pimples and before brushing your teeth apply your spit. Leave for 1 hour and then wash your face.

2. Another good remedy is to grind to a paste equal quantities of neem and mint leaves and apply on the face. Leave on for half an hour and then wash off.

3. Another good remedy is take one-fourth teaspoon each of dry nutmeg powder, sandle wood and turmeric powder. Mix with Camphor lotion and apply on the face. Camphor lotion is made by putting Camphor in a bottle, close the bottle and set in a warm place till the Camphor dissolves

and turns into a lotion.

4. Tamarind pack also helps in reducing pimples. Apply tamarind paste on the face and leave it on for 15 minutes, then wash off. It is a strong antiseptic which clears skin of grease and bacteria in which the pimples flourish.

5. Vitamin A and E capsules if broken and rubbed on the pimples in the night before going to bed also help greatly.

Avoid eating chocolates in any form. Also avoid eating cheese except cream and cottage cheese, shell and salt water fish, very sweet, oily and starchy food because they upset the skin. Take plenty of fruits and green leafy vegetables rich in vitamin A. Vitamin A aids in curing pimples. Besides, Calcium, Zinc and Vitamin E too helps in combating pimples. Constipation puts a brake on the whole system and aggravates pimples. For this reason first thing in the morning, drink a glass of water to which a juice of line has been added. This helps in clearing the blood stream and therefore helps in clearing the skin of its blemishes and at the same time also helps in cleaning the bowels.

■

Hirsutism

Hirsutism is the medical term for a woman who has abnormal growth on the face and body similar to that of men. Adults have two types of hair; vellus and terminal. Vellus hair is soft, fine and colourless whereas terminal hair is long, coarse and curly. Women who have terminal hair on the face and body have high levels of male hormone, an androgen in their blood. Androgen also causes the hair to grow faster and thicker. The primary source of androgen production is the ovaries and the adrenals. Small cysts in ovaries causes them to overproduce androgen. This also causes menstrual disturbances and obesity. Sometimes the victim may also develop masculine characteristics. Some drugs also cause hirsutism. Women who eat too much wheat products are prone to this condition because wheat contains male harmones.

Your doctor will do several tests in order to measure androgen levels. The test will tip the doctor where the problem lies, whether in the ovaries or the adrenal glands.

Do's & Dont's for Hirsutism

Waxing hair causes inflammation and stimulates hair growth by increasing blood supply to the follicles. Shaving is the safest and the easiest methods of temporary removing hair. Contrary to popular belief shaving does not increase the hair growth, it makes it grow faster but one should avoid using blade on the face. Facial hair should always be bleached to make it unnoticeable. But before starting on bleaching, you should keep a few points in mind. When bleaching your face keep the mixture well away from your eyes. Never bleach a pimply face. If your skin is sensitive, apply a little of it on the inside of your wrist to see whether it agrees with your skin. If it does not agree then make your own bleach. To 1 tablespoon hydrogen peroxide add 6 drops of Ammonia. Apply on the face with a piece of cotton wool and wash off after 10 minutes. If you have a dry skin then before bleaching apply a thin layer of cold cream on your face and always bleach under a fan. The other methods of hair removal one:-

1. **Galvanic Tweezer Electrolysis**

   Like needle, expiatory tweezer epilators use electric currents to remove hair. The tweezers grasp the hair close to the skin and applied current travels down the hair shaft to the roots. Pain is lesser than when doing electrolysis.

2. **The Soft Light Laser**

   In this method, first a carbon solution is applied to the skin. The carbon which attracts laser light binds specifically to the hair shaft not surrounding skin allowing the beam to damage the follicle and retard future hair growth. The hair falls out immediately when the area is rubbed with a wet cloth. This treatment gives freedom from hair for 6 months.

3. **The Epilator Treatment**

   First, a cooling jelly is massaged into the hairy areas then the doctor scans the laser over your skin and the incinerated hair fall of within a week. For maximum benefit, you should have 2 to 5 treatments each, one to 3 months apart and you won't see regrowth for a year.

For hirsutism there is no permanent treatment but patients with ovarian or adrenal diseases can be effectively treated. If the patient is obese reducing her weight can reduce the male harmone testosterone levels in the blood. Hormone treatment if done by a good medical practitioner will bring a significant decrease in the growth of hair and definite improvement in the condition within 6 months of treatment.

∎

Beautiful Baby

If you have given birth to a baby girl you should start looking after her beauty right from the time she is in her cradle, for the foundation of beauty is laid in childhood itself. Heredity gives a child the colour of her skin, the basic bone structure and the texture of her hair but the rest depends upon careful nurturing.

If your baby is born with dark fuzzy hair on her face, arms and legs, take 2 tablespoons of gram flour or besan, add a little turmeric powder and cream found on top of the boiled milk. Make into a loose paste and rub this paste gently on the baby's body for a few minutes, then give her a bath. This will not only help remove the superfluous hair, but will also improve her complexion later on.

Massaging a baby's body regularly is of great importance because this gives her strong and flexible muscles later on in life. Through massage you can also improve her facial features, for example if she has a flat nose you can massage the nose lightly with upward movements from the nostrils to the bridge of the nose. If you do this she will have a nice nose neither too long nor too short, but medium and nice. If she has a short and thick neck, make her sleep sometime daily with a thin pillow just below her neck near the shoulders. There should be no pillow under her head.

If she has hairy forehead, you can remove the hair through the gram flour mixture used for removing her superfluous hair.

To get your baby to have lovely pink lips later on in life, every day take a red muslin cloth. Dip it in your milk and rub it on her lips twice or thrice a day. Her pink lips will be the envy of all.

You can also put a few drops of your own milk in her eyes and ears once every week. This way she will have a very sharp eyesight and very good hearing capacity. Later on in life, never apply kajal or anything in her eyes because this will not only give rise to infection but later on it might affect her eyesight also.

If she has scanty hair on her head then rub pure cow's unboiled milk mixed with equal quantity of coconut milk on her head. Leave it on for 15 minutes then give her a bath with baby shampoo.

To keep your baby free from pimples and other embracing blemishes during puberty, after she is six months old, every week take a few drops of neem juice, mix it in little honey and feed her. She will always have a smooth complexion.

From the day she is born clean her mouth with a piece of clean muslin dipped in glycerine everyday. Besides when she is teething never allow her to put anything in her mouth like pencils, rubbers or anything; this will later on give her crooked teeth. For the same reason see that she does not get into the habit of sucking her thumb. Whenever she sucks her thumb, distract her by giving her some toys or you can apply juice of neem leaves on her thumb. The bitter taste will soon make her give up this habit.

When your child is just learning to walk, shoes should be very soft and flexible. Too tight shocs and socks can easily distort a babies feet.

So if you start looking after your baby just when she is born, I am sure she will later on in life make you a very proud mother.

■

Beauty after Twenty

A woman having a perfect, petal-smooth and rosy complexion is the envy of all women. Wherever she goes, heads turn in her direction in admiration; such a complexion cannot be acquired without an effort. It has to be cultivated slowly and gradually by nurturing it carefully from within and without.

Up to the age of 25 the skin is naturally supple, glowing and alive, but it is after the mid-twenties that the skin slowly starts losing its fresh and youthful appearance and acquiring a parched look. This is because the cells deep within the skin layers are no longer able to retain their moisture, and the beauty of the skin mainly depends upon the moisture contained in the cells. The skin, which cannot retain its moisture, turns dry, rough, dull and wrinkled. Therefore, in order to avoid looking prematurely old, you should try to observe a basic skin-care routine after you pass your mid-twenties so that the cells in your skin can retain maximum moisture and your skin remains firm, moist and young right up to old age.

Some people believe erroneously that moisturizing creams and lotions alone will keep the moisture level of the skin in perfect balance. No surface addition of moisture and no man-made lubricant will help you unless you look after the inner life of your skin where beauty and youth really begin.

Therefore, if you want to stimulate your cells to activity for a new look and the feel of youth, feed it regularly with a diet rich in proteins and vitamins B and C. Also, take at least six glasses of water every day, one glass of carrot juice and one pint of either milk or buttermilk. Besides looking after the inner life of your skin, you should also look after its outer life.

It is a good idea to use home-made moisturizing cream regularly after the age of 25 onwards, because this cream helps keep the skin soft, dewy and alive. But before applying any cream, remove all traces of make up with home-made cleansing cream. Foundation cream is not soluble in water and does not come off even with soap. Therefore, a cleansing cream is a must for removing every trace of makeup and grime sooty and coaly dirt. To make the cream take one tablespoon of gram flour and mix to a paste with cream of milk. Stir in a few drops of lime juice and a pinch of turmeric powder. Mix well and apply it with your finger-tips over your face and neck. Leave it on for a few minutes and then rub your face vigorously with your hands. The paste will go on falling as you rub. Remove the clinging paste with hot water, splash on cold water. Blot dry and then apply this home-made cream on the face and neck. Blanch and grind four almonds, one walnut, a couple each of peanuts and charoli to a very smooth paste. Mix in four tablespoons of cream of milk, 2 tbsp. of cucumber juice and one table-spoon each of honey and rose water. Mix well and store in a small bottle. Massage it on the face and neck in circular upward movements, firmly and gently. This cleansing cream should not be just patted on the skin but it should be rubbed hard into the skin so that the oil it contains is picked up by the glands. Leave the cream on for 20 minutes and then wash off. After you cross 25, use only moisture laden foundation creams. Apply little lip gloss on your lip sticks to keep them soft and pretty.

Teenage Beauty

The developing body of a teenager leads to a variety of problems. Some of the most common problems are under active glands, resulting in various skin troubles like acne and open pores and overweight and underweight problems.

If you are overweight (or if this is your tendency), you have to pull out any sweet tooth that you might have and do it immediately. Instead of rich and creamy desserts and sugar-laden drinks, take more milk and eat more nourishing vegetables and fruits. Also, adequate (not giant) servings of meat, fish, poultry and eggs are essential to your health and good figure. But if you are underweight, you must choose foods with high protein and vitamin content. Don't skip meals and don't try to substitute them with quick snacks at odd intervals. That is one of the worst eating habits you can have, which will not help you to round out those angular corners.

Besides taking a proper diet, sleep for at least eight hours daily because the skin cells can only renew themselves while you are asleep.

Exercise in fresh air. Go for long brisk walks both in the morning and in the evening.

During growing years your skin will be getting coarser and the pores will get accumulated with secretion leading to embarrassing bumps and blemishes. To escape this and to keep the skin taut, moist and glowing, keep your skin clean by cleaning it thrice a day religiously. Steam your face at least twice a week. Then, apply a mask made up of two tablespoons dried orange peel powder made into a paste with milk and little rose water. This mask not only cleans the skin but also purifies the pores of your skin so that they function in the way nature intended them to.

Take good care of your hair because this will pay you rich dividends in later years. Brush it nicely both morning and night and if you have reason to think that your hair is falling unduly or looking dull give it the treatment prescribed earlier. And if you have fallen a victim to acne, follow the advice given elsewhere.

As for make up use compact on the face and the palest shade of lipstick available in the market. Apply lip gloss on it if you like. Instead of mascara, brush a little castor oil on your lashes; this will not only give them a wider look but will at the same time encourage their growth. And as for the nail polish use palest of the pink shades.

∎

Beauty at Thirty

When you cross thirty your face undergoes a radical change. The facial skin sags a wee bit, there is also a sign of double chin, the under eye area may look a bit puffy and the first appearance of crow's feet takes place. The neck and hands start showing signs of age. You must not make faces like grimacing, frowning, raising your eyebrows, etc. These actions of the face leave marks on your face which give not only ugly look to the face but leave lines and wrinkles on the face which are not possible to erase. Always treat your skin gently, never drag, pull or squeeze your face.

If you have a dry skin then take 2 to 3 tablespoons of butter or ghee in your diet. Also take vitamin A & E as supplements. Instead of cleaning your face with soap and water, clean with a milk cleanser. Warm 1 tablespoon of oil with 2 tablespoons of milk, put in a pinch of turmeric powder, dip cotton ball in it and clean your face and neck with it, you will be surprised to see that it removes dirt better than any cleansing cream. Rinse your face with water and then apply moisturizer.

But if you have a oily skin then take a diet rich in proteins but restricted in sugar, fluids and salt. Take plenty of fresh fruits and vegetables. Pork and fried and highly seasoned foods should be avoided. Add yeast tablets to your daily diet. This invaluable B vitamin will normalize the oil balance on your skin. Here is a good cleanser for a greasy skin. Put a tablespoon of skimed milk in a cup. Add enough water to create a milky consistency. Apply with cotton wool all over your face and neck. Then remove with facial tissue and blot dry. Always apply moisturizer two to three times a day, this will help to keep your skin smooth and wrinkle-free. Cover your face whenever you go out either with a dupatta or with an umbrella. If you want to protect your skin from ageing and tanning always wear sun-glasses in the bright sun to protect you from lines around the eyes. The skin around the eyes is very delicate, so never rub your eyes unnecessarily. Always apply cream around the eye area very gently. If you have slight puffiness under the eye area then consume less salt and sleep without a pillow. This will not only reduce puffiness but will also stop the formation of double chin. Bathe the eyes upon rising with cold water from the tap. Also apply grated potato on the puffy areas for 10 minutes daily. The puffiness will be reduced. Sometimes anemia gives rise to puffiness. Take iron supplements or foods rich in iron. This will also help in reducing under eye puffiness.

Your feet should look lovely like your face. Wash your feet with linty of soap and pumice stone to smooth away the rough skin. Apply cream or oil after drying them nicely. Trim your toenails regularly and paint your toenails with bright colours. Do not paint the sides of the nails to get a slimmer look.

Like feet you should also take care of your hands. Massage your hands with cream 2 to 3 times daily. The massage movements should be towards the wrists. Give your nails an oval shape and apply light shade of nail enamel to give your hands grace and beauty.

Beauty at Forty

There are very few women who keep on looking beautiful even after crossing the age of forty. These women have cultivated their beauty slowly and gradually through the years and they age gracefully and carry their years as lightly and gaily as flowers in a buttonhole. In later years a slim and trim figure adds as much to the look of youth as a youthful skin.

To keep your body slim, eat a well-balanced diet because after you cross forty. There is a marked decrease in the functional activity of the body. The process of digestion slows down, therefore the fat and the carbohydrate content of the diet should be reduced. Fried and highly spiced foods and junk foods should be reduced to the minimum. Over weight persons need to be all the more cautious of their calorie intake because they are more prone to old age diseases like diabetes, high blood pressure, heart disease, acidity than their slimmer sisters. Therefore, eat more of vegetables and fruits for they are rich in vitamins and minerals and drink at least 1 glass of milk per day and 12-15 glasses of water.

With the onset of age the hair becomes grey but do not pull these grey hair out. Every time you pull out a grey hair, you sow the seed for another few because root at the base of the hair folicale secretes an infectious serum which covers a tiny pinpoint of healthy hair surrounding the white hair and these in turn will go white within no time. If you feel that you must get rid of your grey hair then cut it close to the roots with the help of a sharp scissor. Alternatively you can bleach the offending hair. Just catch it in one hand, dip the cottonbud in the hydrogen mixture, apply on the hair. Let it remain on the hair for 15 minutes, than wash off, this bleached hair will become almost unnoticeable amongst your black tresses. Your neck is a great giveaway. The area can very soon become creepy, lined and wrinkled if you don't pay adequate attention to it. Every day give it the same care and attention you give your face. If you are cleaning, creaming or moisturizing your face continue doing so down your neck. Here is an exercise for maintaining a youthful neck line. Stand straight with chest high and neck tense. Bend head slowly to chest, pulling strongly. Raise your head slowly and repeat with head turned right and then to the left. Do this 10 times. It should be done with easy graceful movements otherwise you will get catch in your throat.

At this age the skin beneath your chin starts wrinkling. Keep your makeup as natural as possible. Use a moisturizer and if you like a little powder.

Go in for soft shades of lipstick and shadows and avoid heavy rimming of eyes with eye-liner. You can use a light coating of mascara over your lashes.

Your food should be light and moisturizing and containing lots of fresh vegetables and fruits. Go easy on fats, sugar, salt and highly spiced and fried foods and junk foods. If you are anemic eat foods rich in iron. Iron absorption is helped by eating foods rich in vitamin C. Calcium is very important for women. Before menopause a women needs 800 to 1000 mgs of calcium per day, but after menopause she needs 1400 mgs per day. The body stores calcium in the bones of the spine till the age of 25 and in the bones of arms and legs till the age of 35. After 35 the stock of calcium keeps on decreasing therefore the older women complain of backache or develop postural defects and even fall prey to fractured bones. You should take plenty of milk and calcium supplements daily.

If you are leading a sedentary life then you should do regular exercise to keep your body fit and healthy. You should walk at least for half an hour daily, and also do some stretching exercises because as you grow older you reduce in height. By the age of 70 you reduce about 2 inches. If you take regular care and attention of yourself you are going to be a healthy old woman, otherwise like many women you will be sick and bedridden.

∎

Beauty at Fifty

Many women look beautiful even when they cross fifty, sixty or even seventy. These women know how to combat the ravages of time.

As you grow older never allow your skin to feel or get dry. Never use soap at this age. You should instead clean your face with a good cleansing milk. Never wash your face more than it is necessary and never wash your face with very hot or very cold water. Always wash it with tap water. In the night massage cold cream into the skin, in the morning before taking your bath, massage Vaseline in the skin. In the day use a moisturizer to prevent any natural moisturizer from being lost to the atmosphere.

Extremely dry or cold weather dries up the skin so take utmost care of the skin during this weather. Mix together yolk of an egg, a teaspoon of cream found on top of boiled milk and a few drops of almond oil. Apply on the face and neck for 20 minutes face. Wash off. Do this at least 2-3 times every week. This will keep your skin supple and smooth. Before going in for your bath take equal quantities of olive, castor, almond and baby oil. Mix and bottle. Massage the body with this oil to keep it soft, smooth and shining.

At this age you get a lot of wrinkles and lines on the face. Lack of moisture and lack of proteins cause these wrinkles. If you do not eat enough proteins, your body uses up stored proteins, the result is wrinkles and sagging of facial and body muscles. Besides proteins, you should drink plenty of water and eat plenty of fruits and vegetables. Once a week take a beaten egg white and mix with 1 teaspoon milk cream found on top of boiled milk and 1 teaspoon honey. Put cotton pads soaked in orange juice over the eyes and apply the mixture on face. Relax in a darkened room for half an hour and then wash off. This will make your skin shine and help get rid of lines from around the eyes and will also make the eyes bright.

Always dress gracefully at this age. Wear saree or salwar kameez. Never follow the fashion of teenagers otherwise you will look foolish. Do not wear gaudy jewellary, go for studs or small hanging eartops. If you are interested in artificial jewellery it is better to go in for various coloured beads rather then chunky metal or plastic jewellery, but you will only look classy and elegant in real or real-looking jewellery.

Try to avoid hair dyes. Hair dyes not only dry the hair but you also start losing hair. With the result you have very scanty hair. If you want you can use henna. If you do not like the reddish colour which henna generally imparts to grey hair then have your hair highlighted. Your salt and pepper hair will really make you look glamorous. As you grow older it is better to have your hair cut short. It is easy to manage. Besides, you look younger. Long hair emphasises the wrinkles on your face, but short hair makes them look less noticeable. Heavily madeup older women look like tarts. For tightening the under chin you should do the following exercise regularly. Push your chin. Go out as far as it will go without following with your shoulders. Now slowly pull the chin inwards towards the throat as far as you can. Relax and do this ten times.

Keep your hair well-brushed, well groomed and well-nourished at all times. This is the time when your skin needs ample amount of grease to counteract the natural dryness of your skin. Every night apply moisturizing cream to your face. In the morning before you take your bath, massage cold cream into your face. Give yourself a facial twice a week. Mix together ¼ teaspoon each of lime juice, honey, cream of milk (cream found in boiled milk) and a few drops almond oil. Massage into the face and neck, leave on for 20 minutes and then wash off. Do not wear clothes and makeup used by teenagers. Wear clothes suitable for your age which will give you dignity and good bearing. Wear light makeup and simple jewellery.

Besides, develop a lively interest in all things and have a sense of humor at all times which will give your face a nice tender look and not a frowning cross look which adds years to your face. Go for long brisk walks. Moreover after 40 you have much more mature and dignified look than before. Therefore, keep your shoulders back hold your head high and above all keep the corners of your mouth up.

Beauty at 60 Plus

Ageing is a process in which many changes take place in the body. The major change comes in the immune system. With ageing, the immune system becomes weak and therefore you fall prey to a number of diseases. The body also goes backwards because of strong rays of the sun, the wind, cold, pollution, drugs, pesticides. All these work in a negative way on the skin making it dry, dull, wrinkled. Besides, the veins and arteries begin to harden making your limbs stiff.

Wrong eating habits, lack of exercise, obesity and uncontrolled mind speed up the ageing process. At 60 plus it is a known fact that almost 80 percent of the people suffer from malnutrition. There are many causes which contribute to malnutrition. Loneliness in old age is one such cause when one is left to himself and finds meal times tedious and boring. The appetite becomes dull and eating good food lessens. Loss of teeth is another cause when eating becomes difficult.

The foods you eat must be rich in raw foods, whole grain cereals, pulses and seeds and should be moderate in proteins. You must take supplements of calcium and Vitamins A, B, C, D & E and minerals like phosphorus and iodine besides of course calcium. These not only prolong youth but also strengthen the immune system and give you zest for life. Eat plenty of curds and you can also eat lean meat, lean fish, eat plenty of fresh green and yellow vegetables and drink milk and plenty of water. Fresh pineapple eaten once a week on an empty stomach improves the skin. Papaya eaten on empty stomach improves the digestion.

At this age the skin turns very dry therefore daily mix a little butter with half quantity of olive oil and gently massage into the skin one hour before taking bath. Always apply moisturizer twice or thrice a day. Every night massage vaseline into the face. Leave on for 20 minutes, then wipe off gently with a tissue paper.

At this age you must try to keep very clean. Many people as they age, they stop looking after their body cleanliness and generally go about unkept and shabbily dressed. But this is the age to look your best, otherwise you will feel most unwanted. Have a real bath daily otherwise you will feel most unwanted. Take a rough towel, lather it nicely with soap and massage it nicely over your whole body. Take bath and apply a perfumed oil in a thin layer over your body, go under the shower for 1 minutes. Wipe yourself dry. Now get into clean and well-ironed clothes.

Teeth should be kept in a very good condition. Brush them twice a day. After you have brushed then clean with a piece of gauze wrapped around your finger to keep them clean and bright.

Your nails should be clean and well shaped. Many older people develop cracks on their feet. Keep them clean by using plenty of soap and pumice stone over them. Finish off with a little oil or vaseline.

Keep the make up as natural as possible. Apply moisturizer and light touch of blush on the cheeks. Use soft shade of lipstick and nail polish but when you go out in the evenings you can apply a bit darker shades.

Keep your hair short and if you do not like cutting them make a plain bun or a simple plait. For special evening you can add a touch of glamour to your hair by putting in a single rose or a gajra.

Walk, dance or swim 3-5 times a week for half an hour.

Practice meditation visualizing an image of yourself feeling healthy, happy and active after 60; the difficulties of failing health are faced by the majority of women but be creative and full of love, understanding and hope. Try to make friends, take active interest in life. Be good, spread goodness. Every day believe in this positive prayer "I am healthy and I will remain healthy and happy all my life".

■

Beat Stress and Rejuvenate Yourself

You have had a grueling day in your office with many more hours to go. Besides you need to look spruced up for that important meeting. Here are some quick ways to beat the stress and rejuvenate yourself.

Dim the lights, dampen a napkin and cover your face with it pressing it lightly around your eyes. Slump into the chair in a relaxed position. Leave arms and legs loose at your sides. Loosen every muscle in your body working from toes to face. Work the relaxation up slowly and stay limp for 5 minutes at the end of which you will feel thoroughly relaxed and raring to go.

Clean your face with facial tissue. Then apply moisturizer all over the face and neck. Then dab on the compact. Run a brush through your hair and apply mascara. Use either automatic roll-on, or liquid or cake mascara. Use the one you find the easiest. They all coat the lashes well. Cover the brush with a light coating of mascara and stroke on the lashes working from the base to the tip. The lower lashes should be tinted with colour. To prevent the mascara from smudging, whenever you apply it on the lower lashes, slip a piece of paper underneath before you paint them. Now take a lip pencil and fill the entire lips by blending in from the edges. To make the lipstick last longer, apply, then blot with tissue and reapply. Apply blusher by smiling and placing colour on the apple of the cheeks using a circular motion. Blend upwards and outwards until there are no lines to indicate where the blusher begins and where it ends. Do not ignore your eyebrows. Comb or at least brush them up with your fingers. If you have scanty eyelashes then take an eyebrow pencil and fill up the sparse areas. The eyebrow should be refashioned by a series of fine lines but never drawn in a solid line.

Perfume should be used as a finishing touch to good grooming. A dainty perfume helps a woman to create an aura of loveliness and appear alluring and attractive always. Use it on the throat, ear lobes, behind the ears, wrist, nape of the neck, temples, inside the crook of the elbows and chest. Perfume applied on these pulse spots stays alive because of the warmth of the skin at these places. The body heat releases the fragrance and you will give out a fragrance wonderfully feminine.

All these sprucing up will not take more than five minutes and then your are ready to go and attend that all important meeting.

Working Woman's Beauty Care

Every other women wants to be a working woman but if you want to work you should look elegant and smart if you want to climb up the corporate ladder.

A working person should always dress formally and must always appear elegant, sophisticated and pleasing to the eye. Wear clothes with vertical lines like straight long skirts which should fall below the knees and slim leg pants which make you appear taller, slimmer and more authoritative. Wear soft pastel shades. For example you can wear soft brown cordory pants with off-white shirt, peach-coloured trousers with black shirt. The shirt should be tucked in with a belt around the waist. Black trousers, with body hugging black coat over white sweater. Sleeveless dark blue top with a long red skirt. Earthen-coloured short sleeved shirt with black trousers. If you would rather go for Indian clothes you can look beautiful and presentable in Salwaar Kameez suits in soft colours. If you would rather opt for a saree then the saree pallav should be pinned up and short blouses and low necklines should be avoided.

Like the clothes, the hair too should be made simply. Either cut the hair short or if you have long hair then you can make a bun. If you have a long face make a side parting and then make a bun at the nape of your neck. And if you have a round face make a central parting and a simple bun at the back. For a change you can also make two buns. Making a parting in the center, twist both the sides of the hair and make small buns on both the sides with pins. For a meatier look put small nets on your buns.

Like clothes and hair, you should have a simple makeup Mix moisturizer with foundation. Blusher should be of a soft shade to give your cheeks a natural glow. Same is true for lipstick and nail polish. Apply a soft matte eye shadow on the eyelids and line your lids with kajal.

Accessories make a great difference; handbags and accessories say a lot about you. Be elegant and smart by cutting out on bangles, big earrings, frills and strappy high heels. Always go in for studs or small eartops. Wear a single bracelet or a bangle and a chain or a thin strand of pearls around your neck. You should have handbag and shoes matching the colour of your dress.

Lastly comes the body language. It is important that you walk with grace with your shoulders back and the head high. Look into the persons eyes whilst talking. Never knit your eyebrows it makes you look nervous and never, never stammer. Dress elegantly and smartly; walk tall and straight, talk and act with confidence if you want to climb the corporate ladder.

Beauty Hints for the Working Woman

Being a working woman you are often invited to parties and outings immediately after work. In short time between work and party how will you manage to look fresh and beautiful. Here are some handy hints if you follow them you will be the cynsore of all eyes without even going home for a change.

1. Carry a few accessories in your bag like mini makeup kit, a few pieces of jewellery and a pair of shoes, or you can keep the makeup kit and shoes in your office in your locked drawer in case of emergencies.

2. Now for the change of dress: just remove the plain blouse you had worn to your office over your saree and wear zari choli or embroidered choli or blouse. Same with churidar Kameez or Salwar Kameez; just lock away your ordinary dupatta and wear an exotic dupatta and see the deference it makes to your appearance. The dupatta and the blouse can make a big difference to the occasion. If you have worn pants or skirt and jacket, then wear under a stripy nicely embroidered and sequined top and in the evening just lock away the jacket and your days clothes will be complete transformed.

3. In the make up kit always carry foundation, lipstick and mascara. Wash the face nicely, then apply foundation all over the face after mixing it with little rose water. Blend

thoroughly with upward outward strokes over the entire face. Mascara is a must for the starry eyed look. If you do not prefer mascara, then you can use eyelash curler. By making lashes turn upwards they appear longer and eyes look larger. Place curler as near to the baseline as possible, squeeze for a few seconds and gently work the curler out towards the end of the lashes for a natural curl. To apply blusher, smile and place a little of your lipstick colour on the apple of the cheeks using a circular motion. Blend upwards and outwards until there are no lines to indicate where blusher begins and ends. For using lipstick, first outline the lips with a lipstick pencil and then fill in the colour with lipstick. For the more natural look, you can use a lip pencil that is either the colour of your skin or a shade darker. Fill the lips with plain lip gloss for a complete natural look. You may also use a frosted lipstick in natural tones, for a party a strong recommendation is to use waterproof lipstick which does not smudge.

4. You can either use a dressy bendi or you can make your own bindi with your lipstick.

5. And as for the ear-rings you can use hops which are latest fad in tinsel town. And lastly do not forget the perfume. While using perfume to avoid wastage and to ensure that it lasts you all evening you should dab it behind your ears and at the pulse points like wrists, inside your elbows, at the end of your neck line and inside your knees. In this way with each pulse beat the perfume will spread further and further not only enveloping you but also everybody else in its lasting fragrance.

Summer Style

In summers to keep cool and composed you require certain things to beat the heat. Here are A to Z of things you should do in summers to keep your cool.

A   Arms : Lovely arms are a tremendous asset. A growth of hair on the arms are a no, no in the hot months. So have them waxed daily. During the bath rub your arms with a pumice stone to keep them smooth and attractive and then pat on a few drops of oil on them.

B   Bathe at least twice daily with an antibacterial soap to keep your body fresh and free from perspiration and body odour.

C   Cotton clothes: Hot season is the season when you should play it real cool. Nylon, georgettes and heavy silks should be stored away and instead you should bring out soft and wispy cottons in the coolest of shades.

D   Dandruff : It attacks your scalp if you do not take a regular head bath. To do away with dandruff mix egg white with lime juice and apply on the scalp. Wash off after 1 hour.

E   Eau de cologne : Chill it in your fridge and spray it over yourself; a wonderful way to keep yourself cool.

F   Fresh green and yellow vegetables : To beat the heat gorge on salads made of fresh green and yellow veggies. Eat them and enjoy a lovely health in this season.

G   For greasy skin: It is the bane of hot season. Drink plenty of water and juices. Avoid fried, spicy and greasy foods. Wash face frequently with mild soap and water. Here is a pack which will help you combat greasy skin. Mix together 1 teaspoon each of grated cucumber, egg white and skimmed milk powder. Apply on the face for 20 minutes and then wash off.

H   Hair : In the hot season the hair too turn greasy if it is not washed regularly. To treat a greasy scalp wash your head with multani mitti. Soak a lump of multani mitti in water. When it softens add juice of 1 big lime. Rub into the scalp and leave on for half an hour and then wash off.

I   For itching : To combat itching in summer apply a paste of baking soda and rose water to the affected areas. Even juice of Tulsi leaves gives relief.

J   Jaljeera : A real must in the hot weather. Chill it and enjoy it to keep your body cool. Now you get the good old jal jeera in tetrapacks also. So instead of colas opt for granny's way of cooling the body with jal jeera.

K   Kness : If you have rough knees take a handful of oatmeal and soak it in milk for 5 minutes and then massage it into your knees. This will make your knees smooth and light in colour.

L   Legs : Since you will be wearing dresses in summer, then you should keep your legs free of hair. Shave them every other day and apply vanishing cream on them whenever you go out to give them a matte finish.

M   Mild calluses : These are thick scaly masses of skin on the feet. In early stages they can be cured by rubbing pumice stone over them in a rotatory motion at bath time. Feet look very ugly when you have calluses and since in this season you are going to wear open shoes be careful about calluses because they always come when you wear ill-fitting shoes.

N   Nails : Oil your nails regularly at night time to keep them in a healthy condition. Remove old nail polish a day in advance to give your nails a chance to breathe in oxygen and to get the advantage of sun and air.

O   Open pores : In not season they become very obvious. The best remedy for them is to rub on the skin half teaspoon of lime juice mixed with one-fourth teaspoon of tomato juice and milk.

P   Pimples : Pimples again become very active due to the greasy skin. The best remedy for pimples is your own spit. The spit found in the mouth early in the morning and at midnight is very poisonous that can kill any disease. Every time you wakeup in the night apply your own spit on the pimples. Before brushing your teeth apply your spit. Leave it on for 1 hour and then wash your face. With in a week you will find great improvement in your condition.

Q   Quiet and rest : Fatigue and emotional disturbances are potential killers of beauty. Specially in warm weather find a cool and dark place and relax.

R   For rash : It is very common in hot weather to get a rash. Sandalwood lotion if applied on the skin once or twice a day gives great relief from heat rash.

S   For sunscreen : It is very important in the hot season. Never go out in the sun without using a sunscreen. It protects you from the harsh rays of the sun thereby protecting your skin from freckles, sunburns and suntan.

T   Tinkling anklets: Tinkling anklets are a part of Indian heritage. Beautiful feet are an asset of which every woman is very proud and what better way is there to show your beautiful bare feet to advantage than by wearing this traditional piece of jewellery around your ankles.

U   Umbrellas : Always carry an umbrella when you are jewellery going out in the hot burning sun, specially when you are going out between 12 to 4 in the afternoon when the sun is at its highest.

V   Very bad breath : In summer or any other season bad breath is a big no, no. You must not eat foods like onions, garlic and radishes. But if you have eaten them to disguise their smell chew cloves, cardamoms or an antiseptic lozenge. Eat curds and parsley. Drink fenugreek or peppermint tea.

W   Withered skin : It is a very rough textured skin full of wrinkles. It is due to over exposure to sum. To protect your skin you must not go out in the sun without an umbrella. Always cream and moisturize your skin after you cross thirty.

X   Exercise : It keeps you going and keeps you fresh and fit. Go for long walks. Jog, run, cycle; do anything but do not be a couch potato.

Y   Yoga : It is the oldest form of healthy exercise which can be practiced in every season. A few moments of yoga a day will purchase for you a toning of muscles and will improve your digestion and circulatory system.

Z   Zest for life: Always be full of happiness and cheerfulness whether it is very cold or extremely hot. It is better to be happy than unhappy because happiness attracts people like bees to honey. There is a well known saying which you should always bear in mind. If you cry you cry alone and when you laugh everyone laughs with you.

■

Be a Winter Beauty

In winters the skin turns very dry, therefore the skin needs extra care and attention. The oil glands just below the surface of the skin become relatively inactive and produce less moisture than usual. This increased dryness of the skin due to the drying effects of the sun and the wind is responsible for causing tiny wrinkles and gives rise to various skin ailments like scaling, itching, chapping and eczema.

1. The best way however to counteract these ailments is to dispense with the use of soap completely. Instead clean your face with milk cream on top of the milk blended with a few drops of lime juice and a pinch of turmeric powder. Every night massage pure Vaseline into your face before going to bed. After bath in the morning massage moisturizer into the skin. If dryness has resulted in scaling take foods rich in vitamins because these vitamins are stored in the fat just below the surface of the skin countering any tendency towards dryness and roughness. Do not eat chilled foods or foods below room temperature. Do not eat cooling things like curds, buttermilk and salads, instead go in for spicy and hot soups. Eat more foods like makai, jowar and bajra and dry fruits and nuts which will provide the much-needed warmth to the body. In winter you should always opt for warm foods which provide the body with warmth and energy so that it does not fall victim to the ailments of

winter.

3. If you fall a victim to itching which is a common complaint during winters then take a tablespoon of sandalwood oil and mix in equal quantity of coconut oil. Apply on the itching parts of the body a couple of times daily to get relief. The juice of tulsi leaves also is equally effective. Another common ailment in winter is eczema. Initially the surface of the skin becomes red but later it turns dry, rough and scaly. Grind a walnut to a paste, squeeze out its oil and apply on the affected parts a few times daily.

4. Winter plays havoc with the hair making it dry, brittle and dull. To bring a healthy shine to your hair take some warm coconut oil and mix it with equal quantities of warm olive oil. Make partings along the hair and dab the oil along each parting with your fingertips. Continue in this way till the whole scalp has been oiled. Then wrap hot towels over the head to keep the scalp as warm as possible. After half an hour when the scalp has absorbed the oil, wash with ordinary shampoo in which one egg has been added; wash the hair in warm and not hot water when using egg on the head.

5. Use a moisturized foundation. On your face touch up your lips with warm creamy colours.

Above all you should eat the right foods to enable your body to fight against the many ills of winter and to put an attractive bloom in your cheeks.

■

ABC of Monsoon Beauty

A   For all round care : Do not get unnecessarily wet in the rain. Even if you get wet and catch a cold, then immediately drink chicken soup. Chicken soup is a very good antidote to cold. When you catch cold you get rough bits of skin on the nose which look very ugly. Rub a little cold cream or Vaseline on the nose and then use a soft piece of toweling material for removing the skin.

B   For building up good bodily resistance : Those who avoid junk food and road side food and cold drinks and eat and sleep well and exercise regularly are generally less prone to monsoon ailments.

C   For communicable diseases : These are ranging from cough and cold to typhoid and malaria. The increased humidity in air plus the unavoidable drenching in the rains gives rise to cough and cold and other rain diseases. As soon as you reach home change to dry clothes otherwise you will not only catch cold but also fungal infections of the skin. Following exposure to rain the feet should be washed in soap and water followed by vigorous massage and a change to dry socks to avoid diseases of the feet.

D   Dark colours : To beat the grey days you should wear vivid vibrant colours. The clothes you choose to wear should not soak up water and should not become limp when they dry and loose their crease. Synthetics like nylon, terelyne, polyester and other man made fibers are ideal for this season because they resist creasing, dry up fast and regain their original shape when dry.

E   Exposure to rain: If the shoes become wet and you are wearing wet shoes, you will immediately fall ill. Always keep an extra pair of shoes at your place of work or in your bag so that you can change into them if your shoes get wet. A good way of drying wet shoes quickly is to stuff them lightly with crumpled newspaper then dry them in the kitchen away from the direct heat of fire.

F   For fungal infection : This usually thrives between toes if you neglect your feet. It causes raw, cracked and itchy skin. It will be cured if you smear the places with alcohol after cleaning and drying them a few times a day. Diabetics should be especially careful of fungal infection otherwise it can lead to serious infection of the feet.

G   Good looks : How are you going to maintain good looks in this humid season? Massage your face with a nourishing cream every night before going to bed. Massage in upward movements and never in downward movements. Twice a week apply this beauty mask on the face. Mix with egg-yolk, 1 teaspoon of orange juice, 1 teaspoon olive oil and a few drops each of rose water and lime juice. Wash off after 20 minutes to give the skin a soft glow.

H   Hairdo : The watch word for hair do should be simplicity. Avoid intricate buns, curls and waves because the humidity in the air will make your hair limp and ugly within no time.

I   Illness: For illness like malaria which is a real nuisance, make a decoration of Tulsi, black paper and jaggery and lime juice and drink while it is still hot. After drinking cover yourself with a warm blanket and lie down. Do this 2-3 times daily to get cured.

J   For jewellery: Monsoons require vivid vibrant colours in jewellery made of gold, precious stones and mina work. Anything which puts a glow in your complexion should be of a deep vibrant shade and apply a dash of Vaseline or lip gloss over it to make them look real enticing.

L   Lines : Pencil your eyebrows in a series of fine lines and never in the form of a thick curved line with one swing of the pencil. The final effect should be a natural looking arch. Use blusher sparingly. Blend it carefully into the skin, see that it is a glow of red colour and not an ugly looking red spot. Finish your makeup with a light puff of powder.

M   Matchsticks : To make your damp matchsticks work, just dip them in your nail varnish and see them light again.

N   Nail varnish : Like the clothes and jewellery your nail varnish should also be in warm colours like glowing turquoise, warm red, deep orange to beat the grey days.

O   Onions : A must in rainy season. A salad made with raw onion, ginger, lime juice and black salt if eaten regularly will help you remain hale and hearty during this season.

P   Prevention: Is the best cure. To avoid falling sick always drink boiled and filtered water, carry your water where ever you go. Do not take chances with outside eatables because you never know if it has been exposed to flies. Flies breed in this season and cause a number of dreadful diseases.

Q   Qaracteristic smell of tulsi plant : It repeals mosquitoes, the carriers of malaria parasites. Juice of tulsi leaves smeared over exposed parts of the body will give protection against mosquitoes and malaria.

R   Raincoat : Brighten up the dull monsoons with a pretty plastic raincoat. Don't buy the readymade rain coat. Get one tailored in a distinctive style. If you like get big patch pockets, a huge collar or a contrasting binding. Select a fairly thick but soft plastic in bright shade with masses of flowers or other designs.

S   Swimming : Swimming should be avoided during this season since several microbes specially those causing colds and conjunctivitis are spread through the pool.

T   Tomatoes : Boil some ripe tomatoes in little water. Strain the liquid and use it to wash your face to remove extra greasiness of the skin during this season.

U   Umbrella : It is no longer something to shelter you from rains. It is a fashion accessory. Choose the umbrella which goes with all your clothes. Do not go for the common colour black. To lengthen the life of your umbrella dissolve 3 tablespoons of alum in water and coat your umbrella with it with a soft towel after keeping it open. Leave it to dry.

V   Very useful tulsi juice : If taken regularly with ginger juice and honey it not only stimulates appetite but also prevents cough and cold, fever and pneumonia.

W   Weight : It is important to keep a constant check on your weight because in rainy season most of us turn couch potatoes gorging on hot bhajias , tea, samosas, halwas and other fattening foods. You can enjoy these once a while but remember to exercise to burn off the extra calories. If you cannot go outdoors then you can walk up and down your staircase a few times. This is also a form of exercise which burns calories.

X   Xtra attention given to your skin : If your face has natural tendency towards dryness, take a yolk of an egg and mix in ¼ teaspoon cream of milk and a few drops of rose water. Wash off after 15 minutes to make the skin soft and smooth.

Y   Yourself : Whether it is raining or any other season you should always enjoy every season and keep your mind lively and try to maintain a cheerful positive disposition.

Z   Zest : Always enjoy every moment God has given you. Go out feel the rain on you face. Get drenched once in a while by walking in the rain and enjoy bhutta (corn - on - the cob) with salt and chili which will put fire in your lips and heart and sparkle of life in your eyes.

SO OUT YOU GO.

How to Make-up

Most of the letters I get these days are about make up. Every teenager wants to know how to apply basic make-up. Today I am going to tell you how to apply basic make up.

1. The first step towards makeup is to have a spotlessly clean face and for this you have to use a cleanser. Clean your face thoroughly with a cleanser and then apply toner on the face with a clean piece of cotton wool.

2. Whether you have a dry, normal, oily or a combination skin there is a foundation specially made for you. For dry skin you get creamy liquid foundations. These contain extra moisturizers to help prevent further dryness of the skin. Normal skin will do either with liquid or creamy foundation. For oily skin use non-greasy cake foundation and on a combination skin use a foundation for normal skin or a shade darker than it. Apply the foundation cobbering all the areas of face and neck. Blend it thoroughly into the skin so that you look natural.

3. Now comes powder which has two uses—one to set the make-up for a long lasting matte finish and two to absorb any shine that appears on the face. Take a clean place of cotton wool and dip it in powder and lightly pat and press the powder all over the face. Flick off surplus powder with a face brush.

4. Fill in the sparse areas in the eyebrows with a brow brush dipped in brown colour. Now go over them with a black eyebrow pencil. Now use the eye shadow. Eye shadow should only be used on the upper lids. Dip the brush in water then take a small amount of colour. Close one eye and place the colour close to and almost touching the lids. Now draw a soft line next to the upper lash line with eyeliner. To draw the line, dip the brush in colour. Hold outer corner of the eyelid taut and draw a fine line as close to the lashes as possible beginning at the inner corner of the eye and finishing just at the outer corner with a light upward turn. To line lower lip take a Kajal pencil with the index finger, hold the lower lid down and away from the eye and draw a line starting at the inner corner of the eye at a point corresponding with the upper line and continue along the lower eyelid just beyond the outer corner slanting slightly upwards as before. Now use the mascara. First brush the lashes downwards to remove any foundation sticking to them then upwards over upper eyelids. Mascara goes better under the fan. The lashes do not gum together due to air. Cover the brush with a light coating of mascara and stroke it on the lashes working from the base to the tips. The lower lashes should be tinted with colour. When the first coat is dry apply the second one. Finally go over the lashes with a dry brush to separate them and to remove excess mascara.

5. Apply the blusher on the cheekbones and see the colour blends well into the skin.

6. Finally apply the lipstick. Fashion the upper lip with a lip pencil start from the outer corner following the natural

curve of the lip and work towards the center. Now draw the line on the lower lip. When the outline is clearly established fill it generously with colour. Now you are ready to take on the world.

∎

Cosmetic Sins

Before we go down to the sins we commit while using cosmetics we should first bear in mind that we should not use anyone else's cosmetics.

They maybe contaminated and you may then fall prey to a variety of allergies which are very difficult to get rid of, or they may not look as good on you as they do on your friends, So never have a hard mentality. Be an individual and be yourself, then only you will look beautiful and attractive. Listed below are some sins while you use cosmetics and instead of looking smart and beautiful you look like a clown. Use the quick fix solutions whenever you find yourself in the situation listed below.

1. **Lipstick on your teeth**

    Solution: Never, bite your lips after using lipstick on them, otherwise with your lips your teeth too will appear red.

2. **Lipstick lines on the cheeks**

    Solution: These usually appear on the cheeks when you keep your hair open, the strands of hair fly all over you while you are traveling and leave unseemly marks on the cheeks. Always tie your hair neatly when you are travelling. You can open them again when you reach your destination.

3. **Smudgy lipstick**

    Solution : This mostly happens when you have a bad cold. Along with wiping your nose, you also tend to wipe your lips with the result the lipstick smudges all around your mouth. When you have cold, try not to apply lipstick. Even if you apply one go for a natural shade so that even if it smudges it does not show.

4. **Half eaten lipstick**

   Solution : This mostly happens when you eat noodles or other oily things in restaurants. Along with the food many people tends to eat the lipstick too. Either eat slowly and carefully or carry a spare lipstick in your purse so that when you finish eating you reapply the lipstick on your lips.

5. **Smudged eye makeup**

   Solution : Use waterproof eye makeup. If you don't have waterproof makeup then stop rubbing your eyes. Pat gently with your handkerchief if you feel itchy around the eyes.

6. **Chipped nailpolish**

   Solution: Use two coats of nail varnish and make sure they cover the sides of the nails which chip first. Also try to buy a nailpolish from a reputed company. These polishes do not chip easily.

7. **Ring around the lips**

   Solution : Outline the lips with a pencil then fill in the lips with a lip brush. Blot dry with a tissue and then apply a second coat.

8. **Streaking foundation**

   Solution: Always add water to the foundation and make it of thin consistency. Apply evenly on the face. Now put on a thin layer of powder. Wet your hands, stand under the fan and pat your face with your hands. Let your face dry. This way the foundation will never streak down your face.

Party Beauty

With the Christmas season almost upon us once again it is the party time, and you need at least 7 days to give your self a glamorous appearance. To look your best for the party season you should exercise and follow a strict diet. Have you wondered why the stars whom you so admire always look so slim and trim with not an ounce of flesh out of place. This is because they follow a strict exercise and diet regime to look honed and toned. Besides exercising and dieting you should prepare yourself a week in advance preceding any big event you have to attend. So here is your preparation plan.

1. Body: Keep it well toned with diet and exercise and drink plenty of water and vegetable and fruit juices. Since it is winter, carrots are available in plenty. Drink at least one large glass of carrot juice every day. Carrot juice helps convert dry and rough skin into silky smooth skin. Besides it acts as a natural blusher which works from within by purifying the blood. Since Christmas comes in the cold season your skin will suffer from the ailments of this season. If your lips have become dry and cracked, then every night before you go to bed apply a thin film of pure ghee mixed with a pinch of salt on them, the hands too turn black and rough. Dip the hands for 15 minutes in warm salted water. Apply a thin layer of Vaseline over them and go to bed. The feet too are affected by the cold weather. Dip feet like

hands for 15 minutes in warm and salted water, apply Vaseline nicely on them. Wear soft socks and go to bed.

2. Hair: If your hair is dry, massage them every second day with warm coconut oil and then wash them with egg shampoo. The last rinse should be juice of 1 lime added to 2 cups warm water. The latest on the hair front is that the hair is becoming shorter, bolder and brighter. Todays young people are going in for razored, layered and textured hair. Straight hair has made a come back and the latest in styling technique is colouring. The most fashionable hair colour is red with purple and orange not far behind.

3. Face: If you have a dry skin, massage the skin with cod liver oil before going to bed. Every alternate day take a tablespoon of strawberries and mix in equal quantity of milk cream (cream found on top of boiled and cooled milk). Apply on the face and leave for half an hour. Remove with tap water. This makes the skin soft and smooth and removes tiny wrinkles. This season the foundations have come out with a glitter, even eyeshadow have glitter in them. Blusher is no longer favored by the rich and the famous, but lipsticks are generally worn in red shades. This is also because of the festive season. Acrylic nails and nail art continue to rule the fashion scene. Gold foil on nails has become very popular and also French manicure. Nail varnish colours have become more metallic and the more adventurous are also using crystals on the teeth. This is the latest fad with the glitterati.

■

Get More

In these days of spiraling prices make the most of your beauty aids. Do you make the most of your beauty aids, get the maximum amount of service from them? Here are some tips worth nothing.

1. Save money by using your lipstick right down to the last remnant in the container by employing a lipstick brush to get to it.

2. If you have a few old lipsticks which are almost over, scoop out the colour with the help of an orange stick and put the colours in a tablespoon. Hold the spoon over a slow fire till the colours melt, then mix thoroughly and pour the mixture in a container. Place the container in the freezer or on a bowl of ice for 15-20 minutes or until the mixture becomes solid, and you have a brand new shade of lipstick.

3. If you happen to have a dark shade of lipstick which is out of fashion, do not discard it. Use it over a white lipstick or better still melt the dark shade along with the white shade and you will have a new soft shade of lipstick.

4. In the hot weather if your lipstick happens to turn soft, keep it in the freezer or on a bowl of ice for half an hour and it will turn hard again. It is a wise idea to keep the cosmetics of all types in the fridge, this way they will last you longer.

5. Do not throw away nail polish brushes. Wash them in acetone then in warm soapy water, dry them and use them as lipstick brushes. If you have a couple of nailpolish bottles in which the nailpolish is dry or nearly over, put in each bottle a teaspoon of acetone, shake well and keep the bottles aside for 24 hours. You will find that the colours have become fluid. Pour all the colours in one bottle fill the rest of the bottle with white, gold, colourless or silver nailpolish. Shake well and you will have in your possession a most unusual colour which will be the envy of all your friends.

6. If your nailpolish spills on the floor. Do not worry, let it dry completely, scoop it up with a orange stick, put it in a bottle, put in some acetone. Shake well, set aside for 24 hours and your nailpolish will be as good as new.

7. To prevent nailpolish from thickening, every week put in a few drops of acetone and shake well. In this way your nailpolish will retain its consistency for indefinite period.

8. A nailpolish bottle top wont stick if a little cream or Vaseline is applied to the threads of the bottle.

9. Do not throw away mascara brushes. Wash them in warm soapy water dry them and use them for brushing your eyebrows.

10. Do not throw away empty perfume bottles. Place them amongst your clothes. Your clothes will have the fragrance of your favorite perfume, but do not keep them in zari clothes, because perfume darkens zari and makes it black. In hot weather keep colognes, scents and your astringent lotion in the fridge. These preparation when chilled can be as bracing as trip to a hill station.

PART - II
BE SLIM & TRIM

Introduction

If you are overweight then it means you are eating more calories than your body needs. On an average you spend 1 calorie per minute but if you want to lose weight you have to burn more calories. Every action of our body needs calories that is energy, but if you eat more than what is required by your body then all the unused energy or calories get converted into fat and is stored in the body. If this reserved store of fat is not used it keeps on accumulating and making the body fatter and fatter day by day. Therefore, if you do not want to put on weight you have to take in less calories than your body needs. This way reserved stock of fat will be burnt by the body and it will maintain its weight. This low calorie consumption is very easy to follow because you are allowed to eat everything provided your total calories consumption remains within the permissible limits. Boiled and raw vegetables have less calories than fried or cooked vegetables. Three big meals a day are more fattening than 6 small meals per day. Rice and wheat have same calorie value therefore it is not fattening. Boiled potatoes are not fattening. Only fried potatoes and finger chips are fattening. Fasting once a week also helps in reducing weight, but if you have any disease consult your doctor before fasting. Besides eating right food you should do regular exercise to tone up your muscles, improve your blood circulation and to keep yourself stress free and happy.

Stay Slim

The word obesity is derived from the latin word "Obesus", which means to eat. Therefore, the fundamental cause of obesity is over-eating. Besides over-eating another important factor is heredity. Children of fat parents are more likely to be fat; it is a known fact that if both the parents are obese then 40 percent of the children born to them are going to be fat, but if both the parents are lean then only 10 percent of their children might become fat.

Obesity starts from childhood. Because of over eating right from childhood, the number of fat cells increase manifold. It is estimated that 90 percent children remain fat when they grow up. During the age of 13 to 16 years it is very easy to increase the fat cells in the body by overeating. If your child is overweight then take her to a doctor to see whether any endocrine disorder is present. If it is not present, then you should train your child to eat less otherwise when your child will reach her adolesence, when personal appearances assume major importance the poor child will become a target of unnecessary teasing. Whatever method you try to be slim you will not achieve success unless you keep down the intake of food. If you think it is worth the effort to remain slim for looks, for health reasons and to please your better half, start dieting from today and establishing new food habits which are low in calories but rich in other important nutrients which will keep your body healthy, happy and slim. You think it is hard? Not at all. Here are a few simple rules which will tell you how to diet the easy way. If you will follow them faithfully, they will surely make you slim in no time.

1. Face upto the fact that the first few weeks of dieting are going to be tough on your stomach because going on a diet means that you have got to eat much less than you usually eat, which means all the time you are going to feel gnawing in your tummy. Whenever you feel the craving for food, that is the time when the "fat" is literally and actually disappearing. So teach yourself to regard these pangs of hunger as the birth pangs of a new you. In the beginning your body will protest, but soon it will stop when it realizes that you mean business.

   In order to train your body to eat less, you must keep busy constantly. If you sit at home doing nothing, naturally you will find that the only diversion you have from your boredom is to eat. Therefore, if you have no work then develop a hobby. Spend the money you usually use to gorge yourself with food on your favorite hobby. Some people who are reducing, find that reading or going to the movies are acceptable substitutes. Other's find substitutes in writing, embroidery, painting, stitching, etc. Once you keep yourself busily occupied, your mind will have no time to dwell upon food.

2. See the calorie chart and substitute low calorie foods for higher ones. Lean meat, fish, chicken eggs, skim milk, cottage cheese, fruits and vegetables are for you. Cut down on heavy desserts except desserts made with honey, gelatin and fresh fruits. But of course you will not like to eat the

non-fattening foods for the first fortnight or so, but slowly and steadily you will develop a taste for them. Once you get used to your new diet, you will reduce by leaps and bounds.

3. For the first few weeks try not to eat with others at the table because naturally the tantilising rich smell of their food will tempt you. Therefore, in the beginning eat by yourself or at a different time from the rest of the household.

4. Take some sort of exercise daily. Go for long brisk walks in the mornings and in the evenings. Play tennis, play with your children, swim and cycle. Do anything but do not keep sitting at one place for any length of time. Keep on the move. This is good for your health and figure.

5. Keep a weekly diary of your weight and essential measurements. Weigh yourself on a reliable scale. Never weigh yourself more than once because the weight varies from hour to hour and the varying measurement of the scale might weigh on your mind and make you depressed. For example, in the morning the weight is normally less than the evening, because your stomach is empty and the fluid which has left the body may weigh a half pound or thereabouts and so you will weigh less for a short time; but in the evenings you will weigh one or two-pounds more. In the same way, the weight varies from day to day because of the varying amount of water the body retains in the different cells and in the bladder. Therefore, a little increase in weight should not alarm you. Weigh yourself preferably in the morning, in the same clothes always on the same scale and on the same day in the next week.

■

Obesity

Obesity is a serious disorder. It can occur at any age and in either sex. It is a health hazard as the extra fat puts a strain on the working of all the major organs of body like the heart, kidney and liver as well on the major joints of the body which bear the bodily weight like hips, knees and ankles. Over weight people fall an easy prey to heart disease, high blood pressure, diabetes, arthritis, gout, liver and gall bladder disorders.

Obesity means extra pounds and these extra pounds put an extra load on your feet and create a disabling pain. Experts note that over weight people suffer higher rates of tendonitis, fractures and sprains than people with normal weight.

Causes

1. The main cause of obesity is overeating. Some people have the habit of eating too much whilst others are in the habit of eating high calorie foods. These people gain weight continuously as they fail to adjust their appetite to reduced energy requirements. Sometimes persons eat because they feel unhappy, lonely or unloved. Some indulge in food because of social or financial constraints.

2. Besides over eating is also due to glandular disturbances like the disease of the pituitary gland wherein an excess of fat is deposited around the chest and the abdomen in a girdle-like fashion. Besides pituitary gland, thyroid gland

too is responsible for giving extra fat to the body. One of the most important function of the thyroid gland is the burning of fat and an underactive thyroid can cause much unnecessary fat deposit all over the body. The hormone secreted which regulates metabolism and burning of fat is called thyroxin and is largely made up of the mineral iodine. Adequate iodine is of foremost importance for normal healthy functioning of thyroid gland. The foods containing iodine are shrimps, oysters, salmon, radish, tomatoes, watercress, cod liver oil and iodized vegetable salt.

These glandular disorders can be corrected by endocrinologists.

■

All About Calories

Calories is a measure of the amount of energy produced by food. Foods higher in calories produce more energy then those with low calories count. By knowing about calories you will find yourself automatically making calorie-conscious choices in food that will give maximum eating pleasure.

To count calories write the amount of ingredient called for in a recipe.

Check up the calorie value for each ingredient in the calorie chart.

Add up all the caloric values to get the total number of calories in the recipe you are eating.

How to cut calories?

To cut down on calories, follow the following methods when cooking. Mostly go in for steamed, boiled and grilled foods; this cuts down the consumption of fats.

1. Substitute skim milk for whole milk.
2. When eating red meat go in for lean meat which contains no fat. Use the young fowl rather than the old hen, the white meat rather then the dark meat, meat without the skin then with the skin. Use only lean fish like pomfret rather then other oily fish.

3. When you want to snack.

   Unbuttered popcorn is only 25 calories per cup.

   Snack on pumpkin and sunflower seeds, get the ones with the shell. It will also force you to eat more slowly.

   Always keep rabbit food around like carrot sticks, cucumber sticks, tomato slices, lettuce, turnips, etc. These have also no calories and are also healthy.

4. Soda has no calories.

5. Cabbage is considered an effective remedy for sliming. It contains tartaric acid which inhibits the conversion of sugar and other carbohydrates into fat. Hence, it is of great value to weight watchers. 2 tomatoes taken in the morning before breakfast is also a safe method of reducing.

6. Eating 2 tablespoons of groundnuts before lunch checks the desire to eat much and therefore helps in reducing.

7. Eating a fresh vegetable salad with lunch also checks you from eating too much because a salad is very filling.

8. Curry leaves too have weight reducing properties.

■

Count Your Calories

For reducing weight, I would suggest 1,500 calories per day and if you can maintain this calorie intake, you will definitely lose weight. But once you have lost weight do not again start gorging on rich and heavy foods which will prove suicide to dieting. Once you have been able to maintain your weight, you can eat the heavier foods like ladoos and rabadi once a week but your calories in a day should not exceed 1,500. With this calorie chart you need not forego anything, but choose things which will give you a sensible, balanced diet.

INDIAN SNACKS AND SWEETS

	Quantity	Calories
Ladoo	40 grams	250
Balushahi	40 grams	250
Imarati	40 grams	250
Rasmalai	40 grams	250
Sohan Halwa	40 grams	250
Badam Burfi	30 grams	200
Pista Burfi	30 grams	200
Jalebi	40 grams	200
Gulab Jamun	40 grams	100
Rasgulla	40 grams	150
Kaju Burfi	30 grams	200

Coconut Burfi	30 grams	200
Kheer	½ Cup	300
Rabdi	½ Cup	490
Kulfi	½ Cup	500
Shrikhand 1Cup	250	
Bread pudding	¼ cup	100
Custard	½ Cup	100
Halwa with milk	1 Cup	930
Chocolate	7 pieces	500

SNACKS

Patties	40 grams	250
Pakoda	1 Cup	250
Kachori 40grams	250	
Bhatura	40 grams	150
Channa 30grams	150	
Samosa	70 grams	150
Dahi Bhalle	1 plate	150
Dosa	1	100
Idli	1½	100
Masala dosa	1	250
Small puri	1	100
Bhelpuri	1 Cup	280
Pani puri	1 Plate	125
Dhokla	1 cup	280
Tandoori chicken	2 pieces	450
Fish Fingers	3	165
Sheekh Kabab	2	300

FRUITS

Fruits	Calories
Medium apple	70
3 medium apricots	55
1 medium banana	55
1 cup cherries	65
3/4 cup currants	55
3 medium figs	90
1/2 medium grapefruit	50
2/3 cup gooseberries	39
1 cup grapes	70
1 medium guava	70
1 wedge melon	50
1 small mango	62
1 large orange	70
1 cup cubed papaya	70
1 cup diced pineapple	75
1 medium pomegranate	90
1 cup strawberries	50
1 large peach	50

VEGETABLES

Vegetables	Calories
1 large tomato	50
2 cuaumbers	50
1 medium onion	50
1 ear corn.	50

1 head lettuce	50
3 small carrots	50
1 cup sliced beetroots	50
1/2 cup shredded cabbage	12
1 1/2 cups cooked cauliflower	15
1 stalk celery	5
1/2 cup cooked green beans	13
3 green onions	13
1 capsicum	15
1/2 cup mushrooms	13
1/2 cup cooked mustard	15
4 small radish	10
1 cup raw spinach	10
1/2 cup cooked turnips	21
1 cup green peas	170
1 cup diced pumpkin	75
1 cup soya bean sprouts	30
1 baked potato	147
Medium boiled potato	83
10 sticks fried potatoes	177
1 medium baked sweet potato	183
1 large boiled sweet potato	246
2 halves candied sweet potatoes	358

NUTS

Nuts	Calories
15 salted almonds	93
1/2 cup shelled almonds	424

6 to 8 cashewnuts	88
2 large chestnuts	28
1 cup shredded fresh coconut	330
2 tblsp. shredded dried coconut	83
15 to 17 roasted peanuts	84
30 pistachio nuts	88
8 to 10 walnut halves	94

DRIED FRUITS

Dried Fruits	Calories
1 cup dried apricots	390
1/2 cup dried currants	268
1 cup pitteed dates	505
4 medium prunes	70
1 cup dried raisins	460

FRUIT JUICES

Fruit Juices	Calories
1 cup fresh or canned apple juice	125
1 cup grapefruit juice	85
1 cup grape juice	165
1 cup lemon juice	60
1 cup lime juice	65
1 cup orange juice	105
1 cup pineapple juice	120
Tomato juice 1 cup	50
1 cup any vegetable juice	36

NON-VEGETARIAN FOODS

Non-Vegetarian Foods	Calories
4 ozs fish	50-60
3 pieces fish fingers 100 grams approximately	150
Hard boiled egg	77
Plain omelete	106
Poached egg	77
Scrambled egg	106
90 grams lamb kidneys	89
90 grams pork kidneys	57
120 grams fried lamb chops	585
4 pieces sheekh kababs	340
120 grams grilled lamb chops	435
100 grams mutton	206
2 slices roasted chicken	215
120 grams boiled chicken	75
90 grams grilled chicken	115

BREADS, CEREALS & BREAKFAST FOODS

	Calories
1 slice bread buttered and toasted	135
1 bun	158
30 grams cornflakes with 1/2 cup milk and 2 tsps sugar	200

1 chapati	100
1 cup boiled egg noodles	200
1 cup cooked macaroni	190
1 cup boiled white rice	200

DAIRY PRODUCTS AND FATS

Dairy products and fats	Calories
1 cup whole rnilk	180
1 cup skim milk	93
1 cup buttermilk	86
1 tbsp. condensed milk	62
1 cup curd from whole milk	207
1 cup curd from skim milk	100
1 tbsp. butter	100
30 grams cheese	115
1 tbsp. vegetable fat	110
1 tbsp. peanut oil	124
1 tbsp. peanut butter	90
30 grams cottage cheese or panner	30

JAMS & SAUCES

Jams & Sauces	Calories
1 tbsp. chilli sauce	15
1/2 cup tomato sauce	80
1 tbsp. worcestshire sauce	10
1 tbsp. orange marmalade.	56

1 tbsp. mixed fruit jam	55
1 tbsp. soya sauce.	8
2 tbsp. white sauce	37
2 tbsp. cheese sauce	65
2 tbsp. chocolate sauce	87

BEVERAGES

	Calories
1 oz brandy	110
1 1/2 ozs dry gin	110
1 1/2 ozs rum	110
1 1/2 ozs whisky	110
3 ozs any type of wine	70
1 cup clear tea	0
1 cup tea with 1 tsp. lime juice	2
1 cup tea with 1 tbsp. milk and 1 tsp. sugar	26
Black Coffee without sugar	0
Coffee with 1 tsp each of sugar and milk	46
1 bottle any aerated water drink.	107
Plain soda	5
Normal bottle of beer	180
London diet beer	85

London diet beer has recently appeared in the market. It is made by the famous company Associated Breweries & Distilleries. This beer has very low carbohydrate content and is extremely suitable for those who are dieting. You will have a mis-conception in your mind that diet beer will have a low alcoholic content. On the contrary the alcoholic content is slightly higher than their other famous brand "London Pilsner" Beer. Besides it is extremely light and still retains the taste and flavour of a normal beer.

■

Weight Control

The major purpose of weight control is to reduce the amount of fat in the body and to increase the amount of muscles. It is in reality a programmed fat control rather than weight control. When we eat, the food is used, stored or discarded. The body stores food, or calories as fat. The less of it we use then the more of it is stored in the body in the form of fat, thus increasing your weight.

Life Insurance Companies are interested in the regulation of weight for the simple and practical reason that they find a definite relationship between weight and mortality. Young people who are underweight and persons over 35 who are overweight have death rates above the average. On the basis of experience, Life Insurance Companies have prepared table of ideal weights which show the lowest mortality rates for various heights which is reproduced below:

Desirable Weights for Men and Women aged 25 and over (in Kilograms by height and frame, in indoor clothing)

MEN (in shoes, 2.5 cm heels)				WOMEN (in shoes, 5 cm heels)			
Height (in cm)	Small Frame	Medium Frame	Large Frame	Height (in cm)	Small Frame	Medium Frame	Large Frame
157	51-55	54-59	57-64	150	43-46	45-50	48-55
160	52-56	55-60	59-65	152	44-47	46-51	50-57
163	54-57	56-62	60-67	155	45-49	47-53	51-58

165	55-59	58-63	61-69	157	46-50	49-54	52-60
168	56-60	59-65	63-71	160	48-51	50-55	54-61
170	58-62	61-67	65-73	163	49-53	51-57	55-63
173	60-64	63-69	67-75	165	50-54	53-59	57-65
175	62-66	65-71	69-77	168	52-56	55-61	59-66
178	64-68	66-73	70-79	170	54-58	56-63	60-68
180	65-70	68-75	72-81	173	55-60	58-65	62-70
183	67-72	70-77	75-84	175	57-61	60-67	64-72

There are certain factors, which may or may not be related to health, such as racial characteristics, body-build, diet, diseases, heredity and social and economic factors that are important influences in determining individual weight and height. In comparing the weights of the individuals of 'light type' with those of small body framework and 'heavy type' with large body and muscular development, a deviation of 10 to 15 per cent from the average weight is usually considered satisfactory.

How many calories to maintain your desirable weight? Daily maintenance of calories.

WOMEN

Weight Lbs	Age 25 years	Age 43 years	Age 65 years
100	1,900	1800	1500
113	2050	1950	1600
117	2200	2050	1750
126	2300	2200	1800
131	2350	2200	1850
143	2500	2350	2000
154	2600	2450	2050
165	2750	2600	2150

MEN			
113	2500	2350	1950
117	2700	2550	2150
128	2850	2700	2250
140	3000	2800	2350
154	3200	3000	2550
165	3400	3200	2700
176	3550	3350	2800
182	3700	3500	2900

The calorie chart is based on moderate activity. If your life is very active add calories, if you are a couch potato, then subtract calories.

When Exercising

A fit figure announces to all and sundry that this is a healthy body. A fit body is always raring to go because it is full of health and stamina which propels you forward with energy which seems inexhaustible. The easiest way to get such a body is exercise. There are plenty of fad diets which promise the earth but nothing really helps except right diet and exercise. Exercise not only keeps you in shape, your skin starts glowing, your body functions at optimum levels, your immunity levels go up, your stamina improves and you do not fall prey to ailments like diabetes, heart disease, stress and high blood pressure. But before launching on your exercise programme please keep these rules in mind.

1. Always do as much exercise as your body permits. Do not overdo it.

2. If you are suffering from any serious disease or if you are a senior citizen then please consult your doctor before doing any exercise.

3. Always wear loose and comfortable clothes. Try to exercise on an empty stomach.

4. Do not exercise in an air-conditioned or a warm room, try to exercise outdoors, if possible.

5. Always do warming up exercises before doing the actual exercises.

The warming up exercises wakes up your body, mobilizes your joints and prepares your muscles for action. Put on your favourite music and do 5 minutes spot marching before embarking upon your exercises.

■

Exercise Therapy

Every woman's best bet for maintaining her health and beauty is exercise. It improves the circulation to the point where areas are stressed and regular exercise will actually develop tiny blood vessels to deliver extra oxygen to the body and remove waste material. Muscles trained by exercise develop greater stores of energy in the form of glycogen. The muscles also grow larger and stronger, lung function improves and heart turns healthier. Somehow we must try to fit exercise of some sort or the other in our daily routine. Forget the car for short trips and walk whenever you can. Stretch when you reach for something on the shelf. Skip elevators whenever you can. Walk up and down the staircase. Park your car a few blocks away from your destination, walk the rest of the distance; do the same for the bus or train. Get off one stop before your destination. Whenever you get a chance stand rather than sit. Do not be a couch potato. Be always on the move if you want to remain young and healthy.

Stretching: This keeps the body firm and graceful. In the morning it awakens the body, during the day it releases tension and stretching at night helps you to sleep. Before you get up in the morning gently stretch first on one side and then the other. Then get out of bed, stand with your feet flat on the ground and reach for the ceiling, try and touch it. Stretch one side, feel the pull from your fingertips to your feet, now stretch the other side. Do this 10 times. Now do the same stretch standing on your toes. Repeat this 10 times then let your body go completely slack.

Cycling: Recent research on heart attacks has shown that cycling is one of the best forms of exercise. It can minimize the likelihood of giving you a heart attack by increasing the blood circulation and exercising all the muscles of your body.

Walking: This the easiest exercise in the world. The act of walking combining both the exercise and the actual striking of feet on a hard surface promotes the addition of essential minerals to the bones. It also works wonders for the circulatory system of the legs and also it improves the entire vascular system. Besides it burns up cholesterol and other fats. But mere walking is not enough, your pace has got to be brisk, because brisk walking though a mild exercise is a good aerobic workout.

Skipping: This exercises the whole body. It strengthens your lungs, legs and wrists. It improves the circulation, firms up the breasts, thighs and buttocks. It tones the muscles, improves your co-ordination, improves your skill at sports, reduces nervousness, increases endurance and helps improve your hand and foot co-ordination. Jumping rope is an excellent means of achieving total body workout. It is equal to jogging 1 and a half kilometers, 350 meters of swimming and half hour of continuous basket ball.

Breathing: Every tissue in the body requires oxygen, therefore practice deep breathing. Stand before an open window and fill your lungs with fresh morning air, then exhale pushing out the last breath. Repeat this for 10 minutes.

The secret of exercise is to develop interest not so much in the exercise but in some hobby which requires vigorous movements of all kinds like swimming, dancing, yoga, karate, tennis, cricket, hiking, gardening, etc.

∎

Spot Exercises

Spot exercises are figure problem exercises that women have difficulty at one time or another. From this article onwards I will tell exercises for the full body and how to maintain it in a healthy and youthful manner. Find out the exercise suited for you and do it regularly for 10 to 15 minutes in order to tone and trim the problem areas.

Arms

Exercise No. 1 ▶

The top of the arms sometimes tends to get flabby. An easy exercise to correct this is to stand with your feet apart in a doorway. Clench your fists and raise your arms high overhead against the door frame. Inhale deeply and press as hard as possible against the frame. Do this 10 times.

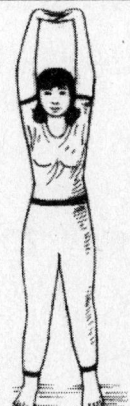

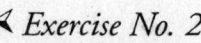

◀ *Exercise No. 2*

Swinging your arms require no energy and is very effective in combating flabby arms. Rotate them first forward and then backwards as high as possible. Do this 20 times.

Keep your hands young

The following exercises will not only keep your hands young but will also help the circulation and you will be surprised to find how these exercises help to alleviate tension and stiffness from your hands.

Exercise No. 1 ➤

Stretch your fingers out as toughly as possible. Relax and then throw them out again. Repeat this 10 times and you will feel all your muscles working.

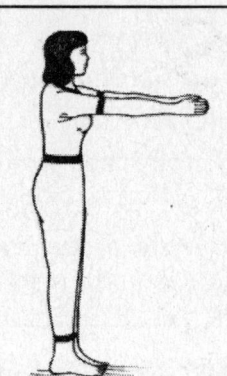

◀ *Exercise No. 2*

Shake your hands until they are completely relaxed and limp.

Exercise No. 3 ➤

Circle your hands from the wrist making the circle as possible and doing four circles to the right and then four circles to the left. Repeat this several times.

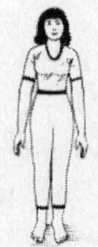 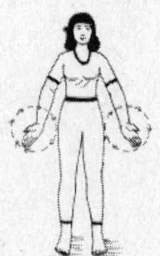

Hips

Excess flesh on the hips is mostly accumulated by sitting down most of the time. If corrective measures are not taken then these fatty deposits may grow quite large and unattractive. In extreme cases, doctors perform surgery known as *lipodystrophia* on this area, but this leaves large scars on the areas, therefore it is always better to do exercise regularly to improve your condition.

> *Exercise* ➤
>
> Lie on your side, head comfortably propped on your palm, which is in turn supported by your bent elbow. Slowly swing your left leg upward as high as it will go, before dropping it down again. Then turn on your left side and repeat the procedure. Continue alternating right side, left side 5 times for each side. The frequent change from right to left creates additional toning as you roll over on your buttocks.

Thighs

Regular exercise is the most reliable way to tone and trim the thighs. Walking is excellent for your thighs and cycling will firm up the slack flesh of the thighs. And if you are housebound then practice cycling by lying on the floor, legs in the air peddling an imaginary bicycle. Here is an exercise which will help you to reduce your thighs.

Exercise ▷

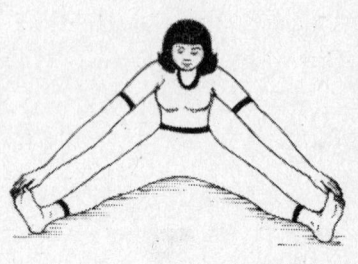

Sit on the floor and extend your legs in a straight line before you. Hold the knees straight and stretch your legs in a fan shape and as far apart to either side as you can. Then very slowly reach for your right foot with your right hand and your left foot with your left hand. You may not reach your feet on the first attempt. So do not force the movements. Slowly return to your original position. Do this 5 times.

Bottom

Bottom is a problem area therefore take care of it before the problem gets out of hand.

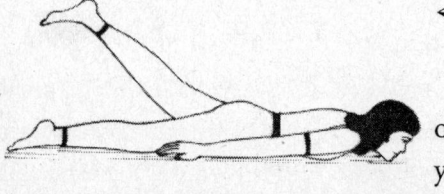

◁ *Exercise No. 1*

Lie face downwards on your stomach with your chin resting on your hands. Lift one leg at a time, keeping your hips on the ground, your leg straight and without moving the rest of your body. Repeat this 5 times with each leg.

Exercise No. 2

Sit on the floor with your legs stretched out in front of you and back straight. Now walk with your bottom forwards and then backwards on music to keep you company. Do this for 10 minutes daily to get results.

Waist

Here are exercises to whittle down a heavy waist.

Exercise No. 1 ▶

Stand upright and clasp your hands tightly over your head. Breathe, display in and out and swing slowly to the right keeping the feet in place. As your arms and upper torso complete a long slow swing around the front part of your body. Continue on around to your left until you have described a full circle. Repeat the circle on the other direction also. Gradually increase the number of times you are doing this exercise till you reach about 5 times a day.

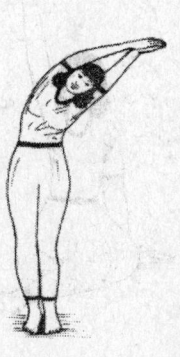

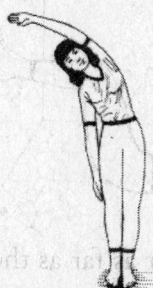

◀ Exercise No. 2

Stand with your feet together, right arm held straight up and left arm easing along your side. Bend side-ways stretching left arm down to your knees and right arm parallel to the floor. Repeat this 10 times on either side.

Exercise No. 3 ▷

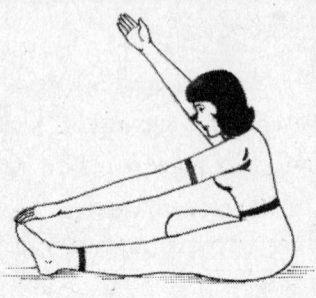

Sit with the left leg stretched out on the ground and the other bent at the knee. Catch the extended foot with your stretched out hand and stretch the right arm towards the ceiling. Do this for 10 seconds and then continue up to one minute. Repeat on the other side also.

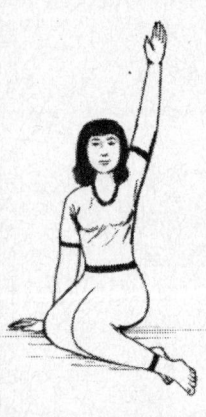

◁ Exercise No. 4

Sit with both legs your folded on one side, keeping knees and feet together. Place right hand next to the right hip on the floor. Lift and stretch your hips while keeping your knees on the floor, look your raised hand. Start with 10 seconds and work up to 1 minute.

This exercise reduces the waistline but also tones up the arms.

Stomach

Exercise No. 1 ▷

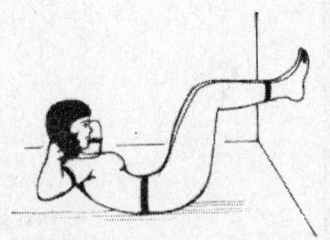

Lie on the floor facing the wall. Bend both of your legs perpendicular and rest the soles of your feet on the wall. Place your hands under your neck and keep your elbows back. Pick up your head, neck and shoulders from the floor as far as they will go and suck in your stomach at the same time.

Exercise No. 2 ➢

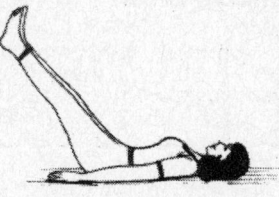

Lie on your back with your feet together and arms by your sides and the small of your back pressed down. Slowly lift your legs to a height of six inches above the ground. Hold this position for 6 seconds increasing it till your muscles get stronger.

Lumpy Knees

Very often you get unsightly lumps on the inner side of the knees. Here are exercises which will help you get rid of these lumps of flesh.

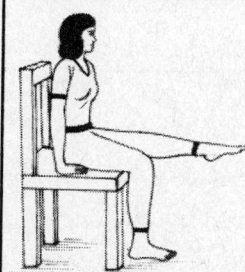

◁ *Exercise No. 1*

Sitting comfortably in a chair stretch the right leg straight before you. Now curl the toes of the foot downward towards the sole of the foot very slowly. Release the toes and relax the leg before repeating the exercise. Do this 5 to 7 times very slowly. Repeat the exercise with the other foot also.

Exercise No. 2 ➢

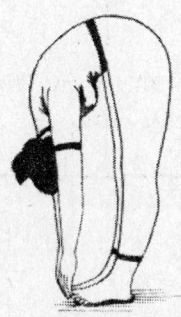

Stand straight, take a deep breath and go up on your toes. Exhale as you bend the knees and lower your body as far as possible. Try to sit on your heels in taking this position. You might need some support in order to maintain this balance. Do this 6 times.

Thick Ankles

If your ankles are thick and seem too big in proportion to your legs then try this exercise.

Exercise

Sit comfortably erect on a chair and hold your feet before you. Describe ten circles with each foot going from right to left. Then reverse the direction and roll your feet in the operation direction. Do this at least 10 times daily.

Calves

For flabby calves do the following exercises to get them back in shape.

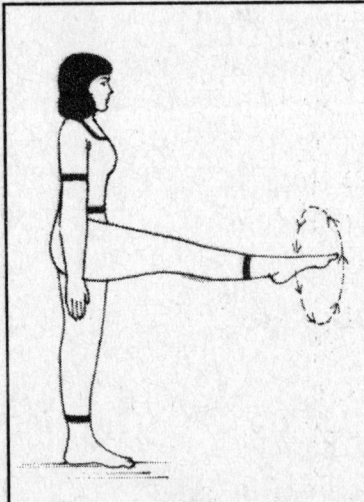

Exercise

This exercise is good both for the knees and the calves. Stand with your legs together and arms relaxed. Raise your left leg, point your toe and stiffen your knee and draw circles in the air with your toes. First clockwise, then anti-clockwise 5 times each way. Repeat with the right foot also.

Legs

This is an excellent exercise to slim and reshape your legs and make them appear youthful and firm. This exercise also removes pain from the heels.

> *Exercise No. 1*
>
> Place your palms on the floor and keep your knees straight. Now take a small step forward with your right hand and then with your left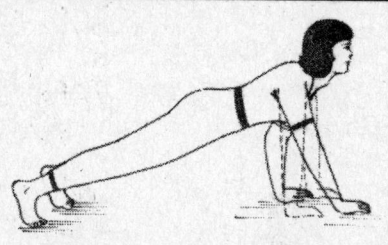
> hand. Then take a small step with your left leg and then with your right. In this manner, take ten steps forward and ten steps backward.

Feet

Here are exercises to relax tired feet.

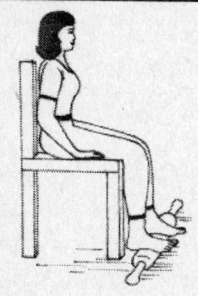

> ◁ *Exercise No. 1*
>
> Be seated on a chair and place a rolling pin on the floor near your feet. Let your feet roll the pin back and forth from the toes to the heels bearing down with a comfortable weight until you feel the increased stimulation in all parts of the feet.
>
> *Exercise No. 2* ▷
>
> Lie flat on the floor with the soles of your feet propped up against the wall. Walk the feet slowly up and down grasping at the wall with wide-spread toes.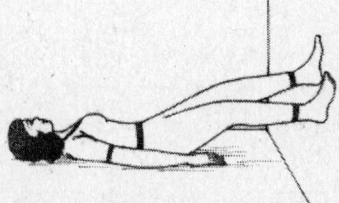
> This open toed movement brings cramped foot muscles into play and activates blood circulation.

Exercise No. 3 ▶

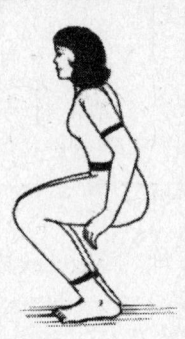

This exercise is helpful in preventing flat feet. Sit in squatting position with your weight on your toes. Slowly rock backwards and come to rest flat on the feet. Slowly roll forwards and rest on the toes. Repeat these movements 5 times. If support is required, hold on to some stable object which will not fall.

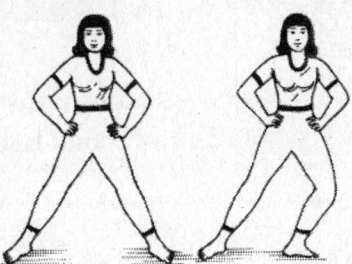

◀ *Exercise No. 4*

This exercise strengthens your toes. Stand with your feet apart and hands at the top of your legs. Bend your right knee and put all your weight at the back of the right foot. Bounce four times and then repeat with the left leg. This exercise should help separate your toes.

Breasts

Women all over the world are concerned about their breasts. They spend large sums of money on drugs, silicone injection and surgery either to increase or decrease the size of their breasts. The answer to a shapely breast lies in exercise and nothing else.

Exercise No. 1 ▶

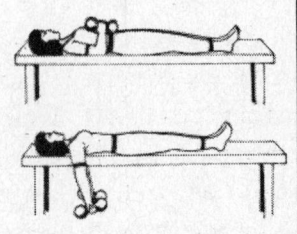

Lay down on a bench with your arms locked over your chest holding dumb bells in your hand. Lower the dumbbells slowly to the floor, then push it to a straight armed position. Do this 10 times. Not only your breasts but even your shoulders and arms are exercising.

Exercise No. 2 ▶

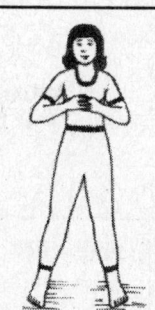

Stand with your arms crossed in front of you. Slowly begin to cross your arms harder until an intense contraction is felt. Start gradually using not more than fifty percent of your effort and gradually build up to the maximum. Breathe deeply before a contraction and you should feel a strong contraction in the pectoral muscles this exercise should be done only two times in a day. If properly performed the above two exercises will give you good results.

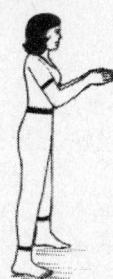

◀ Exercise No. 3

Stand with your feet apart, arms stretched in front of you. Clasp both hands together with elbows bent and press your hands hard against each other hold for count of six. Repeat this 10 times.

Exercise No. 4 ▶

Lie on your stomach, fingers interlocked beneath your chin. Slowly push your head and shoulders off the floor and as far back as possible. Try to keep your thighs firmly on the floor. Count till 5 and return to the original position. Do this 6 times.

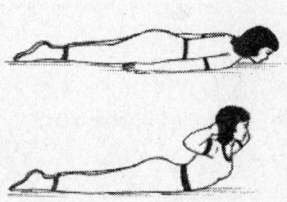

◀ Exercise No. 5

Kneel on the floor with your hands in a prayer position between your breasts. Inhale and press your palms together as hard as you can. Exhale and relax. Repeat to the right side and then to the left side. Do this exercise 6 times.

Whole Body Exercises

Exercise No. 1 ▶

Stand with your legs apart and hands above your head, keeping your knees straight. Circle to the right and then to the left. Try to touch the ground each time. This is a very rhythmic exercise which makes all the body muscles work.

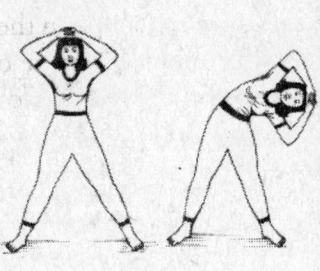

◀ *Exercise No. 2*

Another exercise for the whole body. Lie flat on the floor, arms above your head. Lift up your body bringing your arms out to touch your toes, your head as close to your knees as possible. Roll back gently and lift your legs up to go behind your head into a shoulder. Stand, relax and go down to the starting position. When you master this exercise it is very easy to perform.

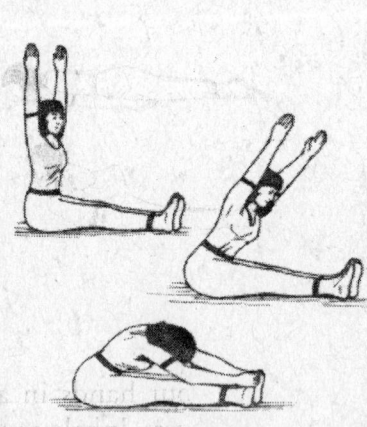

Exercise No. 3 ➢

Lie on your back, heels together feet apart, hands by your side and your chin slightly lowered towards the body. Your mouth should be closed with your tongue touching your upper teeth. Close your eyes and concentrate on the area between your eyebrows or on your deep slow rhythmic breathing. Do this for 10 to 15 minutes.

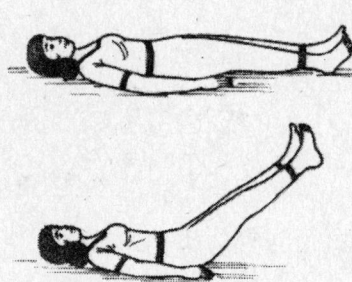

Exercise No 4 ➢

Lie flat on the floor and move your arms and legs in a cycling motion. While doing this laugh heartily. Relax after 5 minutes.

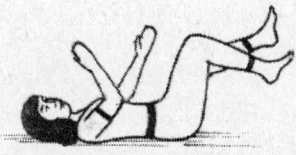

You will gain better usage of your body after performing the above exercises. Daily exercises will give you vast reserves of energy which will allow you to work without feeling tired for long hours.

Light Exercises

Exercise No. 1

Stand straight with both feet together. Bend the upper body first to the left then to the right without straightening up. Inhale while bending the body on the sides and exhale while finishing the circular movement from left to right. Do this five times on both the sides without moving the legs.

Exercise No. 2

Take a light stick and hold it behind the nape of the neck, raise the bar above the head while inhaling, then bring it back behind the head while exhaling. Do this ten times.

Exercise No. 3

Standing, support the right hand on a stick and the left hand on the hip. Raise the left leg straight forward while inhaling and bring it back to the ground while exhaling. Do this ten times with each leg changing the stick in hands.

Exercise No. 4

Stand straight with hands at the hips. Advance the left leg forwards while bending it while inhaling. Bring back in position while exhaling. Do this ten times involving both the legs.

Exercise No. 5

Sit down on the ground with legs separated. Stretch arms on both the sides to the height of your shoulders. With the right hand touch the left foot while inhaling, then with the left hand touch the right foot while exhaling. Do this ten times with each hand. Keep the stomach tucked in whilst doing these exercises.

Exercise No. 6

Lie straight on a bench. Bend one leg after the other bringing each time your knee to the chest. Inhale as you bend the leg and exhale while stretching it. Do this ten times.

Exercise No. 7

Sit on the floor with straight back and legs stretched out in front, hands behind the nape of the neck and the legs joined together. Bend the body forward and try to touch the left knee with the elbow of the right arm. After 6 seconds return to the original position and do the same exercise with the left elbow. Inhale before doing the exercise and exhale whilst finishing the movement. Do this five times on each side.

Exercise No. 8

Lie on the back with your legs joined together. Raise them up as far as they can go while inhaling and bring them back to the ground while exhaling. Do this ten times.

Exercise No. 9

Lie down on your stomach on a flat surface with your hands behind the nape of your neck. Raise yourself as high as possible while inhaling and come to the original position while exhaling. Do this 10 times.

Fun Exercises

These exercises give you fun and enjoyment and at the same time help you to reduce.

Every type of dancing exercises your body and helps you to reduce.

Martial arts like judo and karate also helps.

Roller skating either indoors or outdoors.

Basket ball, tennis, horse riding and cycling are all good exercises. Jumping rope exercises the whole body and tones it up.

Gardening also helps to reduce. Planting, spading, mixing in the fertilizer uses up a lot of calories.

Taking a dog for a walk, not only uses up your calories but also is great fun.

Walk, walk and walk briskly. It costs no money and you can use up to 100 calories in a mile walk.

Warm up with 3 minutes of easy walking. With a little more spring walk at a brisk pace for about 1 minute, then speed walk for 1 minute. At the end of one minute return to brisk pace and then to easy walking. Do this 3 times.

Put on your favorite music and walk around your room for 2 minute at an easy pace. Speed up the pace for 1 minute. Then climb stairs or jump rope for 1 minute. Repeat walk/climb stairs or jump rope three more times. Wind up with 2 minutes of brisk walking.

Facial Exercises

Like the whole body, the face too requires exercising to keep it young and beautiful. By doing facial exercises, you strengthen and tighten the muscles of the face, you stimulate the blood supply and also nourish your facial skin. As you grow older, the muscles of the face begin to sag giving appearance of fine lines called wrinkles. By doing these exercises, you straighten and tighten the muscles and prevent wrinkling of the skin.

Try to push the face out stretching the skin toughly over the skin. Hold it like that to a count of four. Relax and repeat 10 times.

Chin and jaw

1. Lean your head as far as will go. Then open your mouth. Put your chin out and slowly take it up until it closes your mouth. Do this 5 times.
2. Touch your nose with your tongue.
3. Touch the roof of your mouth with the base of your tongue.

Mouth and cheeks

1. Put the forefingers at the corners of your mouth and stretch it as wide as possible. Relax and repeat this 6 times. Keeping the fingers still there, try and pull the mouth shut, forcing the muscles to work. Count 6, relax and repeat 5 times.

2. Open your mouth as wide as you can. Close it very slowly with tension. Repeat this ten times. Turn your head from left to right when doing this exercise to maintain your jaws.

3. Blow out your cheeks as if you were blowing a balloon. Relax and repeat 6 times.

4. With your mouth closed give a big false smile. Relax and repeat this 6 times.

Forehead

Without moving the rest of your face try to move your forehead and without wrinkling it push it up towards the hairline. Hold it to a count of 6 and relax. Do this as often as you can.

Eyes

Open your eyes as wide as possible. Hold to a count of 6 and relax. Do this several times.

Roll your eyes around in a circle. Do it slowly first one way, then the other.

Keep the eyes closed. Contract the muscles by blinking hard. Hold the muscles tight for a few seconds. This reduces puffiness of the eyes.

For dropping eyes, open your eyes, and put your middle fingers into the corners of your eyes, then you gently squeeze the eyes shut and you will feel the muscles there working away.

Neck

Exercise No. 1

Sit with your back straight. Drop your head forward to

touch your chest, bring your head upright and drop it backwards. Do this exercise 6 times.

Exercise No. 2

Sit with your back straight. Drop your head to the right side so that your ear nearly touches the shoulder. Bring the head upright again and drop it to the left. Repeat this 6 times on either side.

Exercise No. 3

Slowly roll the head around front, left, back, right and to the front again. Do this four times first clockwise and then anticlockwise.

Increase Body Activity

Walk whenever possible. Forget bus, train and taxi. Skip the building lift and walk up and down the staircase. Get down a few blocks away from your destination and walk the rest of the way. Whenever you get a chance stand rather than sit. Don't be a couch potato. Always be on the move.

Exercises you can do when doing house work

1. Try to do your own dusting and swabbing. This not only exercises the body but also tones it.

2. Stretch and twist whenever you want to reach for something on the shelf.

3. Whenever you stand up from a chair, grasp arms with feet flat on the floor and push up until you are standing erect.

4. When looking for anything in the bottom drawer of a cupboard or a cabinet, keeping heels flat on the floor, do a deep knee bend. When you straighten up keep your heels flat, let your legs do the work. The same technique should be applied for dusting and making beds that require considerable bending.

5. Whenever you carry any grocery, do not carry the bags in front of you with your shoulders slumping. Hold the bags high, keep the arms straight and shoulders back.

6. Be very conscious of your posture if you want to look slim and trim.

Some Myths about Exercises

1. **Myth:** Exercise increases your appetite, which in turn leads to weight gain.

   Truth: Intense workouts actually suppress hunger. Exercise increases body temperature which discourages hunger. Secondly, exercise decreases blood to the gut and increases the flow to the working muscles there by discouraging appetite.

2. **Myth:** You can eat more after exercise.

   Truth: Eating behaviors has been built up by you over the years, exercises has nothing to do with it. So after vigorous exercise if you eat nothing you are not satisfying your newfound hunger but simply rewarding yourself for doing some exercise.

3. **Myth:** Walking is as good as running.

   Truth: Running or jogging is better than walking. Ten minutes of jogging or running every alternate day is more beneficial then walking. Walking also improves fitness according to doctors.

4. **Myth:** Drinking water between meals leads to indigestion.

   Truth: Drinking water between meals leads to eating less, because water fills you up therefore you tend to eat less. Besides drinking water is good for health, skin and hair.

5. **Myth:** Being a couch potato and overeating increases the waist.

   Truth: More than the above stress plays a major role in increasing the waistline. Researchers at the Yale university claim that evidence suggests direct link between stress and increasing waistline. Stressed women secrete more cholesterol, a hormone which is responsible for increasing the waist and hips. Eating more vegetables and fruits will help you maintain your hips and waist. Quit red meat because they increase body weight. Take vitamin E supplements because these keep body weight in check.

6. **Myth:** Overfeeding a child does not affect his weight, instead makes him healthy and strong.

   Truth : The seed of beauty and body is sowed in childhood. A fat baby will always grow up into a fat girl therefore you should always look after a child's diet right from when she is a baby.

   Get your children to eat a lot of veggies and fruits.

   Teach your kids to eat slowly.

   If they are thirsty give them water and not aerated drinks.

   Do not allow them to snack at any odd time, limit the number of snacks.

   Encourage them to play games like tennis or badminton, volleyball and football. Teach them swimming, hiking and jogging. Exercise and right food will keep their bodies slim and trim.

A Good Posture

Good posture is important for a healthy slim and attractive personality. Posture means straight way of walking with your head held high. With correct posture you will look young, smart and graceful. Bad posture leads to both health and beauty problems. It leads to double chin, heavy waist, sagging breasts and protruding stomach. It also leads to health problems like tired feet, backache, headache and poor digestion.

To maintain a good posture, you must start working on yourself from the moment you wakeup in the morning. When you get up you should hold your head highest as though a string is in the middle of your skull holding it up. Think of your head being kept perfectly balanced by the imaginary cord. If we walk tall and straight, our spine and muscles will carry out the work of supporting our body weight properly. But if we do not walk properly and we walk with a stoop, these muscles have to do the job for which they are not meant. Therefore, people with a slouch get tired more easily than people who walk and stand straight. Besides walking tall and straight we must also learn to sit properly. When we are in a sitting position our spine should always rest against the back of the chair. The shoulders should be straight and the body relaxed. It should never stoop forwards. Legs will look slim and trim if you sit on the chair with one foot slightly in front of the other or crossed at the ankles to one side. Crossing legs at the knees tends to cut off the flow of blood to the legs which may result in painful and ugly varicose veins.

Now we come to the posture of bending and picking up anything from the floor. Do not pick up and lift anything with straight legs. Instead you should try and keep your back straight, now bend at the knees and pick up the thing. But when you are picking up anything heavy, you should keep your back relaxed and your body should be bent forwards so that there is more even distribution of weight throughout the body. When you are traveling by bus, train or ship always stand with your legs wide apart. This way you will not fall even if you are travelling at high speed. To learn to walk tall and straight you can walk around every day for 10 minutes with a heavy book balanced on your head. A good back straightener is to pass a walking stick through the elbows. Hold it lightly across the back. Do this every day for 10 minutes and you will improve your posture considerably. Here is the best posture exercise.

1. Stand straight. Keep the chest raised and the chin in.
2. Draw in your tummy and tuck in your hips so that the hollow in the back is reduced.

Clothes to Hide Body Defects

Bulging stomach

Choose A-line unbelted loose flowing unfitted styles. Try long sweaters and blouses and shirts which make the waistline less noticeable.

Buy skirts which flare at the hemline. Buy hip huggers when buying pants or jeans and wear loose T-shirts or sweaters outside of pants. Avoid short and soft coloured tops which bare the midrif, as they will emphasise your fault. Avoid fabrics which cling to the body. When buying tops, don't buy clothes which are bulky around the midriff and never wear tight clothes or belts.

Heavy legs

Always try to cover them by wearing pants, jeans, sarees and salwars and long skirts which cover the legs. Pants should be straight legged with waist bands, team them with tucked in shirts, blouses or sweaters. If you want to wear a dress keep the hemline just below the knees and wear knee - length boots.

Big breasts

Long jackets and cardigans bring the top and the bottom in proportion. A line silhouettes minimizes the bosom area. Choose tailored unfussy tops and keep to patterns with straight and narrow lines. Choose a bra which gives a flattening shape to your breasts. Don't choose anything which draws attention to the breasts like clinging tops or breast pockets.

Broad shoulders

Give them a soft look with V-shaped necks. Avoid shoulder pads and puffy sleeves, big necklines or bare necklines or halters.

Heavy calves

Wear loose fitting pants. Wear grey or brown stockings with skirts.

Avoid high thin heels. Go in for heels which have enough height to balance the proportion of your legs.

Heavy thighs

Wear pants which are loose fitting in non-clinging fabrics. Same is the case with dresses. Wear salwaars and sarees. Wear skirts with soft gathers and pleats. Do not wear any dress which hugs the hips. Do not wear any top which ends at the broadest portion of your thighs.

Heavy hips

Wear a long blouse over a slim skirt. The hips covered with a long blouse makes the hips look slender. Do not wear fitted blouses and short fitted jackets.

Wear semi-sheer blouse over a camisole and slim trousers to conceal large hips. You can also wear blouses cut exactly to your hip size with deep side slits. This shape looks very flattening on big hips.

Gently flared hips or wrapped styles conceal large hips. Stay away from shorts and go in for knee length or above the knee culottes with slight flares. The length of the garment is very important for large hips. If you are short, wear calf length skirts and tall girls can wear skirts up to ankle levels.

■

Colours and Textures for Obese People

There are very few people who have perfect figures. The whole art of dressing is to create an optical illusion that emphasizes the good points and minimizes the weak points. It is here that colours and textures are important if a person is on the heavier side.

When choosing fabric for yourself, keep in mind that bulky and heavy fabrics will add width to the body. Soft and clinging fabrics will hug the body and reveal the silhouette. Shiny and glossy fabrics will increase your size because they reflect light. Dull surface and medium weight fabrics tend to give slender appearance. As they do not have highlights, they tend to minimize size and conceal the outline of the silhouette. Prints and patterns should be in proportion to the size of the figure. A large orient on a small figure looks ridiculous. In the same way a small print on a large frame will look absurd. Therefore, overall prints should be small and not contrast too much.

To look slim, stripes must be narrow. Bold broad stripes will make you appear broader. Vertical lines create an optical illusion that help you look taller and slender than you really are. When the eye moves in upward direction it gives an illusion of tallness and thinness. When the upward motion of the eye is interrupted by cross wise lines then the object looks shorter and rounder. Besides fabrics and prints select a colour to suit your weight. If you are stout, dark coloured fabrics will make you appear stouter, therefore you should go in for cool colours like blues and greens that tend to recede and make you appear slimmer. Light colours make your figure seem much larger than dark ones. You should use medium colours that blend with the background but do not necessarily define the outline of the figure. For example, you should choose a forest green colour instead of muted grape colour, instead of royal blue a soft rose and instead of bright pink grey.

■

Make-up Secrets

Over weight is not only reflected in the body but also in the face. Glowing and shining hair combined with healthy smile adds to the beauty of even a very obese face. An obese face can look and appear beautiful if you learn the art of hiding the defects like round cheeks, double chin and heavy jaws with right make-up tricks.

Always apply make-up on a very clean face. Therefore first clean the face with a good cleansing milk, wash it well, pat dry.

If the skin is oily then apply astringent and if it is dry them apply a good moisturizer to the skin.

Use light and dark foundation to slim down and reshape your face. Use light foundation in the areas around the eyes and below the eyes to hide dark circles and also on blemishes. On this apply a dark foundation with damp sponge nicely so that it blends completely with the light foundation.

Puffy cheeks

Create a hollowness under the cheekbones with a darker foundation, extend it to the jaw line blending all the time into the skin.

Double chin

Use a dark shade right under the chin with a lighter shade in the crease on either side. For a fuller broader double chin, apply shading just under the jaw bone. Blend from ear to ear along the jaw line and under the chin.

Broad nose

To slenderize nostrils, apply lighter foundation over the entire nose and then apply darker foundation on either side of the nostrils. For too broad nose apply two strokes of dark foundation down each side.

Lips

To apply lipstick properly, you must learn to use the lip brush effectively. You should avoid dark lipsticks and use softer shades. Before applying lipstick, apply foundation to the lips because this makes a good base for the lipstick and at the same time it blots out the natural lip line so that you can outline a prettier shape with your brush. Fill the brush with colour, fashion the upper lip first with your lips slightly apart. Start from the outer corner following the natural curve of your lips and work towards the center. Let the tip of the brush draw the line on the upper lip. Use the side of the brush on the lower lip working at one half of the lip at the same time. When the outline is clearly established fill it with colour.

Thick lips can be made to look thinner by painting them within the natural lip line and covering the remaining area with foundation cream. If the lips are thin, the upper lip can be extended above the natural lip line but care must be taken to see that the extended portion follows the natural curve of the lips. The lower lip should be full and well-shaped by extending the lip line a little below the natural line of the lower lip.

Your focus should be on the eyes; learn how to use eye shadow and mascara artistically. Eye shadow gives an enchanting touch of depth and mystery to the eyes. Eye shadow should only be blended on the upper eyelids. Use dark shades of shadow sparingly. Try mauves, pastel greens and blues instead. Close one eye and place a small amount of colour to and almost touching the upper eye lashes from inner to outer corner of the eyes. It should then be blended with your index finger or brushed upwards into a fade way effect below the eyebrows. It should be darkest near the lid.

Mascara

First brush the lashes downwards to remove any foundation sticking to them then upwards over the upper eyelids. Apply mascara with a clean brush. Cover the brush with a light coating of mascara and stroke it on the lashes working from the base to the tip. The lower lashes should be just tinted with colour. When the first coat dries, apply a second one. When the second coat also dries, go over the lashes with a dry brush to separate them and remove excess mascara. If properly applied the lashes should be a series of individual hairs and not one solid mass. Remember your eyebrows. They should be well-shaped, therefore always have them shaped from a reputed beautician. For puffiness under the eyes, before applying foundation, use a concealer or a lighter foundation.

You Ask We Answer

1. **Do drugs and pills help in losing weight?**

   It is very dangerous to take drugs and pills for reducing weight; they are very harmful and sometimes they may even turn fatal.

2. **What about surgery to remove extra fat from the body?**

   Operations to trim fat from hips, abdomen, arms and breasts are being performed but they are difficult, expensive not always successful and can sometimes prove life threatening.

3. **Does massage help in reducing?**

   Massage does not help in reducing, it can only tone the body and help the massager to reduce and not the client because the massager is exercising himself while massaging the client.

4. **Does sweating and sauna help?**

   These are temporary methods which help remove extra water from the body which is quickly replaced when you drink water or any liquid. These may prove harmful by putting undue strain on the heart and blood circulation. Sauna is especially harmful to the body because it raises the body temperature to high levels and also the pulse rate.

5. **Are new fad diets helpful?**

   They are not advisable because they encourage rapid weight reduction in very short time. Doing without this or that food or having only this food or that food will not meet body's need for balanced nutrients which may result in dangerous diseases.

6. **If I do not eat my regular three meals a day will I then lose weight?**

   Our body requires calories continuously throughout the day, so if you skip breakfast or lunch, the body takes away valuable stored proteins from the body instead of fat to fulfill its energy needs. So if you do not eat the whole day, in the night instead of 200 calories you will consume 1000 calories, so the extra calories will turn into fat and the body loses valuable proteins and puts on fat.

7. **When should a diet control be started?**

   Diet control should be started as soon as a child becomes obese. The fat cells are always present in our body, but as the child grows the number of fat cells increase, so an obese child is more likely to grow up into an obese individual, therefore a fat child should be treated immediately, just like a fat adult.

8. **What are the benefits of dieting?**

   After weight loss, a patient naturally starts looking and feeling better. Since the weight loss in dieting and exercising is slow, steady and systematic the skin does not sag so that there are no stretch marks and wrinkles. The patient's health also improves dramatically.

9. **Is exercise as important as dieting?**

   Yes both go hand in hand. Without exercising, dieting will not help you.

   Our food gives us a large amount of calories. It is very important that we burn up the extra calories through exercise to obtain optimum health, that is, we should strike a balance between the calory intake and output.

10. **Besides reducing what other benefits does exercise gives?**

    Exercise depresses the release of stress-related chemicals and keeps the blood pressure normal. It also increases the efficiency of the heart. It helps in burning extra calories and lowers the blood sugar and helps in controlling diabetes by stimulating the secretion of insulin. Deep breathing exercises improve the vital capacity of the lungs and reduces the incidence of allergic diseases like asthma.

    The bones become strong and the risk of falling prey to osteoporosis is greatly reduced.

    The muscle tone improves and the muscles become strong.

    Exercise speeds up metabolism and increases oxygen supply to the brain. This has a mood elevation effect.

    ∎

Combat Bad Eating Habits

Daily new fad diets appear in the market offering an easy cure to the weighty dilemma of numerous obese people. But the diets almost always fail because they do not change a persson's eating habits. To really succeed you must count your calories and keep a record of what you are consuming throughout the day. You will be amazed that not many people are consciously aware of their eating habits. If you keep a careful record of each morsel you put in your mouth you will be amazed to see the results. You must understand the basic eating habits you have and then you will be able to solve your weight problem.

Here are some of the questions you must answer and write down to find out your bad eating habits and then improve upon them. Do you eat whilst working in the kitchen, whilst cleaning the house, feeding the dog or watching TV? Do you eat fast? People who eat fast take in more calories than people who eat slowly. When you are in a hurry, you will gobble food without realizing how much you are eating and therefore you are overweight. Therefore before you eat, look at the food, thank god for the delicious food he has put before you and then take your food, eat slowly, chew thoroughly and enjoy your food. Cut the food into small pieces and eat one piece at a time. In this way you will not only enjoy your food, you will also eat less, keep down your weight and say goodbye to acidity and flatulence. Do not load you house with food. If your fridge and kitchen is loaded with food, it is but natural that you are going to be tempted to eat it. Try to keep low-calorie foods in the house so that even if you are tempted, your food does not give you added calories.

Most of the time food is eaten when you are alone and bored. So try to keep yourself occupied with some hobby or pastime which takes your mind away from food. Last but not the least write down a schedule of what and when you will eat that day and stick to it. If you have scheduled lunch for 2 on a particular day do not eat the meal before 2 even if you are hungry, you can eat rabbit food till that time and nothing else. This together with exercise will surely keep your weight down.

■

Distract Yourself from Food

Take up a hobby or a pass time. Learn computers, candle making, beauty courses, painting, singing, dancing. Infact anything which keeps you busily occupied and takes your mind off food.

Go out of your house and go window shopping. Check out on new things and places. This will not only provide you with a nice exercise but will also make you aware of the new things happening around you.

Go to the park or the garden. Have nice long walks and meet new and interesting people.

Get rid of the accumulated junk in your house. You will be surprised at how much stuff you have collected over the years.

Try to find ways to put the junk to good use, either recycle or find somebody who will take it from you.

Make friends, reach out to people and see how they welcome you. But do not expect too much from a friend and you will be happier.

Try new styles and make-up tricks. Keep occupied with looking better and better still.

Start comparing yourself with your slimmer friends. A little competition will take you to the road of success, but too much rivalry will turn exhausting. You must always remember that there will always be someone more beautiful and slim than you are but you can always strive to be personally the best and for this you have to use all your energy to stop over eating and start exercising.

■

7-Day Menu for Reducing

IST DAY

Breakfast

First thing in the morning take 1 cup warm water to which strained juice of a lime and 1 teaspoon of honey has been added.

or

Take 50 grams raisins and soak whole night in 1 cup water. Next morning crush them with a spoon and add the juice of a sour lime.

Either of the above concoction taken first thing in the morning helps in clearing the blood stream and therefore clears the skin of all its blemishes and at the same time helps to work the bowels.

Later on for breakfast take 1 cup skimmed milk. 1 thin slice of bread. Spread with 1 tsp. butter. 1 poached egg. To poach the egg fill a small katori with lightly salted water. Bring to a boil and then reduce heat. Break the egg in the water. When the white is firm carefully remove the egg with the help of a slotted spoon. Then take a fruit like apple, orange, peach, apricot, grapes, berries or pomegranate or a slice of any melon or grape fruit or pineapple. Besides, take 1 fish liver oil capsule like Elasmin pearls for vitamin A & D, 100 miligram vitamin C tablet and six brewers yeast tablets containing the entire B family.

Lunch

Poached fish, 2 melba toasts, finger salad.

Poached fish

2 slices pomfret. 1 carrot, scraped. 1 onion peeled. 1 stalk celery. 1 bay leaf.

Salt and pepper to taste. Place fish in a pan and cover with boiling water. Add the rest of the above ingredients and cook till the fish is fork tender.

Melba toast

Lay 2 slices of bread on a shallow baking tray, place tray in a slow oven and bake till perfectly dry and crisp. Spread each toast with half teaspoon of butter.

Finger salad

Fix a plate with the following vegetables : tender carrot and cucumber sticks. White and red radish, small whole tomatoes and onion slices and shredded beetroots, shredded cabbage and turnips. Season with salt, pepper and lime juice. You can also add shredded spinach or lettuce. You needn't have all the vegetables mentioned above but try to eat as many as you can.

Teatime

1 glass tomato juice.

Dinner

2 cups vegetable soup, grilled liver, spinach bhaji, 1 chapati.

Vegetable soup

1 medium onion, peeled and sliced, 3 medium sized tomatoes, peeled and quartered, 1 stalk celery sliced, 1 medium potato, peeled and sliced, 1 medium carrot, scraped and sliced. 1 small turnip, peeled and sliced, salt to taste.

Place the vegetables to cook in 6 cups water along with salt. When the vegetables are cooked nicely puree part of the mixture at a time in an electric blender at high speed. Eat with a pat of butter and reserve the remaining soup for the next day's lunch.

Grilled liver

Take 1-¼ inch thick slice calf liver.

Brush the liver slightly with peanut oil and sprinkle with salt. Place on oiled griller and grill not longer than 4 minutes on either side. Sprinkle the top with a little chopped parsley and green onions.

Spinach bhaji

½ cup chopped spinach, 1 small onion, 1 inch piece ginger, 1 green chili, 1 tomato, Salt and chili powder to taste.

Put the spinach to cook with all the above ingredients. When it is tender, mash. Reheat before eating.

If you like a dessert over your dinner then take a fresh fruit like apple, orange, a slice of grapefruit or pineapple, etc.

Bedtime

1 cup skimmed milk.

2ND DAY

First thing in the morning drink the warm water, lime juice and honey mixture. Later on take 1 soft boiled egg, 1 slice of bread spread with half teaspoon of butter. And anyone of the fruits mentioned on the first day's breakfast and all the tablets mentioned therein.

Lunch

Braised lamb chop with vegetables. 1 chapati. 1 glass buttermilk. Mixed vegetable salad. 100 grams grapes or strawberries.

Braised lamb chops with vegetables

250 grams lamb chops from lean mutton, 1 tomato, 1 onion. 1 carrot, 1 turnip. Salt and pepper to taste.

Fry mutton to a red colour in 1 tbsp. peanut oil in nonstick pan. Then cover with hot water and cook till the mutton is almost done. Put in the vegetables and continue cooking till both the mutton and the vegetables are cooked. You can vary the vegetables according to your personal choice.

Mixed vegetable salad

Mix together finely sliced raw carrot, beetroot, cucumber, spinach and tomato and sprinkle over with lime juice, salt and pepper.

Teatime

Take ½ cup of spinach juice mixed with 1-1/2 cups of carrot juice.

Dinner

Left-over soup from previous day's dinner, curried meat balls, 2 toasts spread with half tsp. butter each and fruit sponge.

Curried meat balls

250 grams ground lean mutton, 1 small onion minced, ½ inch piece ginger, minced. 1 tbsp. cornflour, 1 small egg. 1 tbsp. soya sauce, 1 tbsp. fine dry bread crumbs, 1 tsp. sliced parsley. ½ cup skimmed milk, 1 tsp. each of powdered cumin seeds and coriander seeds. ¼ tsp. garam masala. Salt and chili powder to taste.

Combine together meat, salt, chili powder, onion, ginger, cornflour, egg, soya sauce, bread crumbs and parsley. Shape into round balls. Heat 1 tbsp. oil in a non-stick pan and fry the balls to a nice brown colour. Put in milk and the remaining spices and cook for 15 minutes. Check occasionally and add a little more milk if necessary.

Fruit sponge

¾ cup orange juice, 1 tbsp. gelatin, 4 tbsp. sliced fruit of your choice, 1 egg white stiffly beaten, 2 tbsp. honey.

Dissolve gelatin in 1 tbsp. hot water. Add the juice and honey. Warm the mixture till honey dissolves. Then add fruit and chill. When partially set, mix in the egg white and chili till firm. Decorate with orange slices.

Bedtime

1 cup skimmed milk.

3RD DAY

Breakfast

Take warm water, lime juice and honey mixture. Besides, take 1 scrambled egg, 1 slice bread spread with 1 tsp. butter, 1 cup skimmed milk and 1 fruit of your choice. Also take all the vitamins as shown in the breakfast of the first day.

Scrambled egg

Beat egg with 1 tbsp. skimmed milk and scramble in non-stick pan in 1 tsp. oil. If you want to add any vegetables like mushrooms, capsicums, etc. then lightly sauté the vegetables first.

Lunch

Fish curry, raita, 1 chapati, salad as shown in the lunch of 2nd day's menu and 1 orange.

Fish curry

2 slices pomfret, 100 grams mixed vegetables like peas, french beans, carrots and cauliflower, 1-inch piece ginger, minced, 1 tbsp. curds, 1 small tomato, 1 small onion minced, ¼ tsp. each of turmeric powder and garam masala, a few coriander leaves. Salt and chili powder to taste.

Apply salt and turmeric to the fish and set aside for 15 minutes. Heat 1 tbsp. oil in non-stick pan and fry ginger and onion. Add tomato and curds and cook till dry. Put in the vegetables, mix well and cover with hot water. Add fish and cook till both the vegetables and fish is done. Sprinkle coriander leaves and garam masala on top.

Raita

1 cup curd made out of milk with cream removed, a few inner heart leaves of cabbage, ½ tsp. roasted and powdered cumin seeds, 1 green chili, minced, ¼ inch piece ginger-minced, 1 tsp. sugar. A few springs coriander leaves. Salt to taste.

Mix together all the above ingredients.

Teatime

1 cup each of carrot and cucumber juice.

Dinner

Hearty non-vegetarian delight, 2 melba toasts, dried fruit compote.

Hearty non-vegetarian delight

1 chicken leg without skin, 1 egg, 1 slice pomfret, 100 grams mixed vegetables like French beans, peas, cabbage carrots, etc. Salt and soya sauce to taste.

Beat the egg lightly. Steam the vegetables and fish. Flake the fish and chop the vegetables. Boil chicken in 2 cups of water. When tender, strain out the soup and soya sauce into the egg and stir well. Mix in the rest of the above ingredients.

Dried fruit compote

Take 100 grams of dry fruits like prunes, apricots and raisins. Cover them in warm water and 2 tbsp. honey. Keep them in the fridge for 24 hours before eating.

Prepare melba toast as shown in the dinner menu of the first day.

Bedtime

1 cup skimmed milk.

4TH DAY

Breakfast

Take warm water, lime juice and honey mixture. Besides, take 1 egg omelete. 1 slice bread spread with 1 tsp. butter, 1 cup skimmed milk and 1 fruit of your choice. Also take all the vitamins as shown in the breakfast of the first day. To make omelete take 1 egg, 2 tbsp. sliced cream cheese. 1 tbsp. sliced tomato. Salt and pepper to taste.

Beat the egg with salt and pepper. Pour egg into non-stick pan, add cream cheese and tomato when the underside is firm, turnover and cook till the otherside is firm also. You can make an omelete in the non-stick pan without oil but if you want you can add a teaspoon of oil.

Lunch

Cheese delight, 1 roti, Salad as shown in the lunch of second days menu. Pudina raita.

Cheese delight

Prepare cheese: take ½ liter skim milk. ¼ cup curd. 1 tblsp. lime juice.

Boil the milk and mix in curd and lime juice. When the milk curdles strain through a cloth, tie it loosely and hang it up to drip in a bowl until no more water flows. Then place the cheese between 2 flat plates and place a heavy weight on the uppermost plate for half an hour. Remove the weight, plates and cloth and cut the cheese into small pieces. Besides take 1 cup fenugreek leaves. 1 chilli, minced. 1 medium tomato, sliced, a few coriander leaves, ¼ tsp. turmeric powder, 1 tsp. coriander powder, a big pinch gram masala, salt and chili powder to taste.

Heat 1 tsp. peanut oil and put in all the spices, leaves, tomato, chili and coriander leaves. When the leaves are tender, mix in the cheese and remove from fire.

Pudina raita

1 cup curd made of milk with cream removed, Handful of mint leaves. A few raisins, ½ tsp. cumin seeds, salt and chilli powder to taste.

Grind mint, cumin and raisins to a paste and mix all the above ingredients together.

Teatime

1 glass carrot juice.

Dinner

Moong dal delight, vegetable stew, 1 roti, curd fruit cup.

Moong dal delight

½ cup whole moong sprouted, ¼ cup curd, 2 carrots, boiled and sliced, ¼ coconut, grounded, 1 small onion, 2 green chillies. 1 tsp. each of mustard seeds and coriander powder. ¼ tsp. turmeric powder. Salt and chillies powder to taste.

To sprout the moong, soak in water for 14 hours. Drain and tie them in a clean wet cloth. Set aside for 24 hours at the end of which the moong will develop sprouts. Grind onion and chillies to a paste. Heat 1 tsp. peanut oil and add mustard. When the seeds stop popping add the onion and fry lightly. Add dal, turmeric, salt and 2 cups water. When the dal is cooked, mix in the rest of the above ingredients. Eat only half, keep the remaining for the next day's lunch.

Vegetable stew

250 grams mixed vegetables like French beans, carrots, cauliflower, peas and lady fingers. 1 big tomato, 1 tsp. grated ginger, 2 green chilies, ½ tsp. each of turmeric powder and cumin seeds, a few coriander leaves. 1 tsp. coriander powder. Salt and chili powder to taste.

Heat 1 tsp. peanut oil. Add cumin seeds and ginger. When the seeds stop popping, add all the spices, chillies, coriander leaves and tomato. When the tomato turns soft, add the vegetables and 1 cup water. Do not put lady fingers with other vegetables. Put them in when the other vegetables are almost cooked.

Curd fruit cup

Put alternate layers of sliced fruit and chilled curd in a fruit cup. Dribble the top with honey.

5TH DAY

Breakfast

Take the warm water, lime juice and honey mixture. Besides, take 1 scrambled egg, 1 slice bread spread with 1 tsp. butter, 1 cup skimmed milk and 1 fruit of your choice. Also take all the vitamins as shown in the breakfast of the first day.

Lunch

Moong dal delight as cooked in the 4th day's dinner menu. 1 roti, drumstick bhaji, finger salad as prepared in the lunch of first day. 1 fruit like orange or apple.

Drumstick bhaji

2 drumsticks, scraped and diced into pieces, ½ tsp. grated ginger, ¼ tsp. cumin seeds, A big pinch each of turmeric powder and garam masala, 1 medium tomato, sliced. 1 tsp. coriander powder, Handful of coriander leaves. ¼ cup skimmed milk, 1 tbsp. tomato ketchup, salt and chilli powder to taste.

Heat 1 tsp. oil and toss in cumin seeds and ginger. When the seeds stop popping, put in tomatoes and all the spices and cook till soft. Add drumsticks, milk, ketchup and salt and cook till soft and almost dry. Sprinkle coriander leaves on top.

Teatime

1 glass carrot juice.

Dinner

Cream cheese bhaji. Vegetable soup as prepared in the first day's dinner, 2 toasts, apple delight.

Cream cheese bhaji

Prepare cheese as shown in the lunch of 4th day's menu. Besides, take 1 big tomato. 1 chilli, minced, a few coriander leaves. ¼ tsp. turmeric powder, 1 tsp. grated ginger, a big pinch cumin seeds, 1 tsp. coriander powder, salt and chili powder to taste.

Heat 1 tsp. oil and put in the cumin seeds and ginger. When the seeds stop popping, add tomato along with all the ingredients with the exception of cheese. Cook till dry. Add 1 cup warm water, put in the cheese and cook for 5 more minutes.

Apple delight

1 tsp. butter, 1 shredded apple. Honey to taste. 2 finely sliced almonds.

Heat butter till it melts. Put in apple and heat thoroughly. Sprinkle with honey and almonds.

Bedtime

1 cup skimmed milk.

6TH DAY

Breakfast

First thing in the morning take either warm water lime juice and honey mixture or raisin mixture. Later on take 1 egg omlete, 1 slice of bread spread with 1 tsp. butter, 1 cup skimmed milk and any fruit of your choice. Also take all the vitamin tablets mentioned in the first day breakfast.

Lunch

Green chana bhaji, mixed vegetable raita, 1 roti. Vegetable stew as shown in the dinner of 4th day's menu. 1 fruit of your choice.

Green chana bhaji

1 cup boiled green grams, 1 cucumber, sliced thinly, 1 small potato, boiled, peeled and diced, 1 small onion, shredded, 1 tsp. sugar, 1 tbsp., lime juice. A few each of sliced mint and coriander leaves. Salt, chilli powder and pepper to taste.

Mix all the above ingredients together.

Mixed vegetable raita

1 cup curd made of milk with cream removed. 50 grams mixed and finely sliced vegetables like peas, French beans, carrots, cauliflower (steamed), 2 green chilies, ½ tsp. roasted grounded cumin seeds. A few sliced mint and coriander leaves. Salt and chili powder to taste.

Mix all the above ingredients together.

Teatime

1 cup pineapple juice mixed with 1 cup beetroot juice.

Dinner

Mutton stew, 2 toasts, orange sponge.

250 grams lean mutton. 100 grams mixed vegetables like tomatoes, carrots, peas and French beans. ¼ coconut. A few each of mint and curry leaves, 1 small onion, 1 tbsp. coriander powder, ¼ tsp. each of turmeric powder and garam masala. Salt and chilli powder to taste.

Grind coconut and extract juice. Set this thick juice aside. Put 1 cup warm water in squeezed out coconut scrapings and set aside for 15 minutes, then squeeze out the milk. This is known as the thin milk. Put mutton, salt and spices in this thin milk and cook till almost tender, put in the vegetables and mint leaves and continue cooking till both the vegetables and the mutton is tender. Fry onion and curry leaves in half teaspoon of peanut oil to a light brown colour. Put over the mutton and serve at once.

Orange sponge

1 cup orange juice. 1 tbsp. gelatin. 2 tbsps. honey.

Dissolve gelatin in 1 tbsp. warm water. Also dissolve honey in orange juice by placing both on slow fire. Mix in gelatin and chill.

Bedtime

1 cup skimmed milk.

7TH DAY

First thing in the morning take either warm water, lime juice and honey mixture or raisin mixture. Later on take 1 poached egg, 1 slice of bread spread with 1 tsp. butter, 1 cup skimmed milk and any fruit of your choice. Also take all the vitamins mentioned in the first day's breakfast.

Lunch

1 roti, cream cheese delight as prepared in the lunch of 4th day's menu, 1 glass buttermilk, vegetable stew as prepared in the menu of the 4th day.

Teatime

1 glass tomato juice.

Dinner

Chutney fish, marrow treat, 2 slices of bread, baked apple and carrot delight.

Chutney fish

2 slices of pomfret, 2 pieces of plantain leaves.

Chutney: A small piece of coconut, handful coriander leaves, 2 green chilies, ¼ tsp. cumin seeds, 4 mint leaves, 1 flake garlic, small onion, lime juice, salt and chili powder to taste. A big pinch sugar. Grind the chutney ingredients to a paste. Coat each piece of fish nicely with chutney. Roll the fish up in plantain leaves. Tie with a piece of thread and steam the fish for 10 minutes on either side. In the absence of plantain leaves use well-greased brown paper.

Marrow treat

1 cup sliced marrow or pumpkin. ¼ cup pureed tomatoes, ½ inch piece ginger minced 1 green chili minced. 1 small onion, minced. Handful of sliced coriander leaves. Salt and pepper to taste.

Heat 1 tsp. peanut oil and fry cumin seeds. Then add ginger, onion and chillies. Cook till soft. Mix in the rest of the above ingredients and cook till thick. Mix in 2 tbsp. skimmed milk and remove from fire.

Baked apple and carrot delight

1 medium apple, grated. ½ cup shredded carrot, ¼ cup grated coconut, 2 tbsps. honey, 1 tbsp. butter, Dash of salt, ½ tsp. cinnamom, ½ tsp. lime juice.

Mix all the above ingredients together and put in a greased ovenware glass dish. Bake in a preheated moderate oven for 25 minutes.

Bedtime

1 cup skimmed milk.

HEALTH 🌳 HARMONY

Health Harmony is an imprint of **B. Jain Publishers (P) Ltd.**, which is a 35-year-old publishing house. Our books are very popular for two reasons. Firstly, the prices are very reasonable and secondly, the quality of material and content is excellent.

Tree in the **Health Harmony** signifies Holistic life and that is what the mankind should aim at. This tree is lush green which signifies total health. Also, its roots are well fixed to the ground which motivates us to be down to earth and respect our roots. Thirdly, this tree is in harmony with its atmosphere i.e. air, water, soil. This helps us to understand that we have to preserve our environment if we have to remain healthy and in harmony.

Our publishing house conceived the idea of Health Harmony two years back to provide interesting and top-quality reading material for seekers and believers of health and holistic living.

Under the banner of **Health Harmony**, we have expanded our collection to encompass Health, Sprituality, Astrology, Feng Shui, Vastu, Palmistry, Numerology, Management, Career & Travel related books. Till now, we have added more than 400 books to our **Helath Harmony** collection. We were the first to publish books on Reiki, Tai Chi, Acupressure and books by Rudolf Steiner who is a great European Philospher.

It is our endevour to provide to the masses of Indian Subcontinent (India, Pakistan, Bangladesh, Nepal, Bhutan, Sri Lanka, etc.) the best published works of the world at low price without compromising with the quality of the books.

One of the main reason for the popularity of **Health Harmony** books with the readers is that these are written by authors who are authority on the published subject. Like some others publications, we do not encourage compilation and cut-paste work.

For Free Catalogue details refer overleaf

www.bjainbooks.com

FREE CATALOGUE COUPON

Yes, I am interested in Health Harmony titles. Please rush me the catalogue.

FREE CATALOGUE ORDER FORM
(Write in Capitals)

Name ....

Complete Mailing Address ....

....

....

....

.... Pin ....

Ph. (Res.) .... Ph. (Off.) ....

E-mail. ....

Date ....   Signature

Mail this coupan to

HEALTH 🌳 HARMONY
an Imprint of
B. JAIN PUBLISHERS (P) LTD.
1921, Chuna Mandi, St. 10th Paharganj, New Delhi-110 055
Ph.: 3670572, 3670430, 3683200, 3683300
Fax: 011-3610471 & 3683400
Website: www.bjainbooks.com, Email:bjain@vsnl.com